The Ancestral Indigenous Diet

Achieving Native Health in a Modern World

by Frank Tufano

The Ancestral Indigenous Diet:
Achieving Native Health in a Modern World

Copyright © 2019 by Frank Tufano

All rights reserved. This book or parts thereof may not be reproduced in any form, stored in any retrieval system, or transmitted in any form by any means — electronic, mechanical, photocopy, recording, or otherwise — without prior written permission of the publisher.

ISBN: 978-1-7344306-1-5

Editorial services by Jared Wade, 86 Sixty

Published by Frank Tufano, United States of America

First printing edition, 2019

Frank Tufano
www.frank-tufano.com

Table of Contents

Chapter 1
Rediscovering Our
Ancestral Indigenous Diet

Chapter 2
Creating My Diet:
Frankie Boy's Journey to
Optimal Health

Chapter 3
The Fundamental Four:
The Nutritional Foundation of
the Ancestral Indigenous Diet

Chapter 4
The Other Nutrients:
Understanding and Getting
Everything Else You Need

Chapter 5
Chronic Inflammation:
How to Avoid the Silent Killer

Chapter 6
Plant Food Myths:
Why Fruits, Vegetables, and
Grains Aren't Necessary

Chapter 7
Food Quality: The
The Biggest Factor in
Nutrition and Health

Chapter 8
Food Sourcing:
What to Eat and How to Get It

Chapter 9
Food Preparation:
Cooking and Eating to
Maximize Nutrition

Chapter 10
Understanding Natural Hunger:
The Three Types of Satiety

Chapter 11
Frequently Asked Questions (FAQ):
Addressing Common Ancestral
Indigenous Diet Concerns

Chapter 12
Beyond Nutrition:
Water, Sleep, Sun, Exercise,
and Modern Problems

Chapter 13
Eating As Nature Intended:
Your Journey to Optimal Health

Chapter One

Rediscovering Our Ancestral Indigenous Diet

Have you ever seen a wolf wear glasses? Are gorillas making kale shakes in the jungle? Are sharks wearing braces?

Humans are animals. We evolved into our current physical form tens of thousands of years ago before spreading out across the globe. We look, live, and eat differently depending on the specific location where we settled. Every aspect of human physical development has been guided by these factors over hundreds — even thousands — of generations. Not only was our development dictated by these factors, but many of the problems of modern civilization are a result of us having abandoned this environment.

The largest change in recent generations has been to our diet, although other critical elements of health — water, exercise, sun exposure, and sleep — also undergoing major shifts.

The human diet, all across the planet, has always been composed of high-quality animal and plant foods that vary by region. According to some [historical accounts](), indigenous people didn't suffer from the modern degenerative diseases that are so common today, let alone dietary conditions like type 2 diabetes.

My belief is that this was primarily due to what they ate. Their water was also free of modern contaminants, both physical and chemical, and they used to get much more sun exposure while staying active throughout the entire day. Now, after spending most of our waking hours inside, we try to make up for hours and hours of sedentary activity with a small window of exercise then we sleep poorly, surrounded by blue light from electronic screens, before waking up to an alarm clock in the middle of our sleep cycle.

There is no going back to the past. Few would want to. But with a little bit of effort and a change to our mindset, we can take some steps to rediscover our ancestral health. There is direct action that you can take right now — primarily by adding high-quality animal foods to your diet — to begin repairing the damage caused by modern eating and lifestyle choices.

Only one thing is stopping us: What we've been told all our lives.

The Ancestral Indigenous Diet vs. the Paleo Diet

Some people familiar with diet trends may think they have heard this before. Isn't this the Paleo Diet? Certain elements of my approach to nutrition do line up with the Paleo Diet, and some of the ancestral-based concepts are similar. But, no, my philosophy is quite different.

At its core, the Paleo Diet focuses more on what foods you *can't* eat as opposed to foods you *should* eat. Many civilizations have consumed grains that didn't exist in the days of cavemen, for example, and lived in excellent health nevertheless. Dismissing this knowledge — just to devoutly follow the idea that we must eat exactly like our ancestors before the Agricultural Revolution — can begin to border on religious.

Instead, we need to dig deeper and begin to understand which foods are bad for us and which are absolutely critical. Recognizing which foods are most important from a nutrient, vitamin, and mineral standpoint is largely absent in most Paleo Diet descriptions.

Paleo, in many ways, is about restriction. My Ancestral Indigenous Diet, above all else, is about prioritizing the foods that you must consume.

For me, nutrient density is the basis of everything. We start by understanding which nutrients are the most essential to health and focus all of our attention on consuming them. Then, at the same time, we cut out everything that doesn't serve a clear purpose.

Yes, it does turn out that most of the best foods to consume are similar to what cavemen survived off of. But the argument for why we should eat them now in the 21st century is based much more in nutritional science — not dogma and modern marketing spin. Even more importantly, the Paleo Diet has been largely corrupted by people who started making brownies with 30 different "paleo" ingredients, not to mention the corporate and special interest groups working to make sure people don't understand the importance of food quality.

I'm not bashing the Paleo Diet from afar. I have tried it and understand why Paleo has appealed to so many people. The version I followed involved me eating five pounds of sweet potatoes per day in an attempt to fix my lack of energy. My skin turned orange from all of the beta-carotene, and I looked green in certain lighting.

It was actually pretty fitting. I looked like an alien — because I was eating a diet that isn't realistic on this planet.

Eating Like a Carnivore

If I am speaking against sweet potatoes, does this mean I think meat is the only path to health? Is this the Carnivore Diet, another recent "fad diet" in the world of nutrition?

Yes — but also no. Very much no. Some of you may be familiar with me identifying as a carnivore through my YouTube channel. And although my dietary regime does fall under carnivore , there are far more pieces to this puzzle. This is mainly because the Carnivore Diet, at least as it has been popularized over the past few years, is incomplete and lacks nutrition.

Many medical professionals are skeptical of the Carnivore Diet and have warned people not to jump on this trend. While some of their worries — about missing grains and veggies — are unfounded, they are correct to wonder how someone eating only steak can be healthy.

For those who are not familiar, let me offer some quick background. The Carnivore Diet hit the mainstream in 2018 and has been growing steadily in popularity ever since. A lot of this is thanks largely to its association with Canadian psychologist Jordan Peterson and his daughter Mikhaila Peterson, who touts her meat-only lifestyle for curing a range of health problems she had been dealing with for years.

For Mikhaila, and as it is usually described, the Carnivore Diet's primary benefit is reducing inflammation and working as an "elimination diet" that cuts out any problems you might have with food allergies or intolerances. (Almost nobody struggles to digest meat.) It also cuts out sugar and most carbs, which fits in with the Keto Diet push that has gone even more mainstream and generally makes people feel better than the energy spikes and crashes of the Standard American Diet (SAD). Compared to the aptly named SAD way of eating, it is no surprise that people usually feel better after going Carnivore.

And unlike another trendy movement, the Vegan Diet, the Carnivore Diet is not entirely void of key vitamins and nutrients. But the people who preach eating grain-fed steak all day, every day, are missing many essential things as well. Throw in all the hormones, antibiotics, agrochemicals, and other negative substances rampant in conventional meat, and I understand why doctors are against it.

My diet is much different. The food prescribed by the Ancestral Indigenous Diet does come almost entirely from animal sources. So it does overlap with the carnivore way of eating (as well as the Keto Diet). You can call it carnivore. But it will not match up — at all — with the popular version of the Carnivore Diet you will find online or at the bookstore.

Besides, there actually are some plant foods that are fine to eat and a few that offer legitimate nutritional benefits. If you decide to consume them, options like wild blueberries, macadamia nuts, and avocados are the lesser of the evils. Seaweed contains iodine and electrolytes.

These plant foods, however, are not necessary to achieve optimal human health. Still, some people like to eat them — whether for culinary or other reasons — and I will help explain why some plant foods must be avoided while others can provide some supplemental benefits without many drawbacks.

So, in short, no, this is not the Carnivore Diet that you may have heard about. It is very, very different, even if it shares the concept of exclusively sticking to animal products.

The Ancestral Indigenous Diet is more about teaching you the principles, handed down by those who survived and thrived throughout history, that will help you achieve true natural health.

Some of this is non-negotiable. You must consume certain vitamin-rich foods. But there is also a lot of flexibility. I will not be forcing you to follow some 30-day meal plan. I won't dictate exactly what you need to eat.

Instead, this book will show you *how to eat* in a way that you can follow forever.

The Power of Meat

Paleo, Carnivore, Vegan, Vegetarian, Keto, Mediterranean, Atkins, South Beach, Raw, Primal, Local, FODMAP. Today, these diet terms are all discussed constantly throughout traditional media, social media, and the YouTube community.

There is simply far too much contradicting information about diets. Doctors push statins to lower cholesterol. Well-meaning wellness advocates adopt a plant-based diet to avoid heart disease. Keto dieters push electrolyte consumption and high fat consumption from junk food.

Most people agree that fruits and veggies are good for you. But has anyone actually questioned why? Or even argued for the opposite? There is so much to analyze and interpret — with so many conflicting studies — but one thing is for certain: the presence of high-quality animal food and high-quality plant food in every native diet. Remember that term: high-quality. It is what I advocate above all else.

There once lived communities in modern-day Switzerland, for example, that consumed mostly rye bread and raw grass-fed cheese, supplementing with meat and milk. Some Australian Aborigines ate hundreds — even thousands — of wild plants and animal foods. Certain groups of Native Americans in North America got more than 80% of their calories from buffalo. Even in modern times, there are so-called "blue zones" (the term for places with unusually high life expectancy) that incorporate both high-quality animal and plant foods as the basis of their diet.

The exact animal and plant foods eaten by different native groups varied widely. There were, however, two consistent factors in all of these communities: the presence of animal foods and a level of food quality that is rare today in the United States.

And it is the vitamins specific to these animal foods — the essential fat-soluble vitamins — that are the key to human health. There is no other source of these nutrients that is present in all regions of the world at all times of the year.

Upon inspecting the nutritional profile of plant foods, we see that they actually lack certain nutrients found in animal foods. Many have a high "paper value" of vitamins and minerals. But the "bioavailability" of these nutrients is very low in reality, primarily because we cannot utilize the nutrients in these plant foods as effectively as those from animal sources.

This is compounded by the presence of "anti-nutrients" that serve as a defense mechanism for fruits in vegetables. Not only that, but some people are genetically unable to convert the vitamins found in plant foods into the form that is needed in the body. (One key example is the conversion of the beta-carotene found in vegetables to retinol, the animal form of Vitamin A.)

Even people whose bodies can make the conversions require fat for the vitamins to be metabolized correctly. And where is the only place you can acquire fat as all times of the year in all places on earth? Animal foods. Fat access from plants is very limited to specific parts of the world that naturally produce the few sources that do exist (like avocado, coconut, and other nuts).

The fat phobia pushed over the past half-century by the Western medical community — and with the full support of the agricultural industry — has made people forget about this. Maybe more than protein (and the lean chicken people now devour), fat has always been the foundation of the human diet. Nothing else offers the same combination of nutrition and caloric energy.

Even the media and mainstream medical community are starting to acknowledge that fat and cholesterol are not bogeymen, although certain entrenched groups continue to resist. This is a nice baby step, but they continue to miss the message on the essential nutrients unique to high-quality animal foods.

In our modern world of abundance, people have grown disconnected from the natural world. But the caloric density of plant foods is very low. This alone makes it clear why animal foods provided the only viable source of energy for tens of thousands of years throughout human evolution — not to mention all the labor required to gather low-calorie wild plants. It's no wonder people opted for grains once the Neolithic Revolution hit and agriculture became viable.

In the big picture, widespread access to fruits and vegetables is a relatively modern concept. And we should recognize that many indigenous groups were in perfect health while effectively only eating animal products and wild grains. So, when creating our modern diet, the safest assumption is that we need to focus on obtaining our nutrition from animal foods. Plants, including grains, should be afterthoughts. We aren't surviving in nature any more. We get to pick and choose what we eat. And if our ancestors had a choice, those tribesmen would have always picked the hunt over the farmer's plow.

Unlearning Assumptions and Conventional Wisdom

Many people find these ideas difficult to consider. Assumptions based on conventional wisdom may never be overcome. Cultural norms are such a strong tool, and food pyramid pseudoscience has become ingrained into our society. Combined with fear-mongering, propaganda, closed-mindedness, and pride, these preconceived notions may forever continue to prevent people from rediscovering their true, ancestral, natural health.

Meat is bad for you. Fruit and whole grains promote health.

This is what public health officials and medical authorities have been telling Americans for the past century. But even as we are learning more and more that this isn't true — through both scientific research and individual experience — people continue to, quite literally, take this message to their grave.

If something isn't working, it is time for something new.

But in the case of the Ancestral Indigenous Diet, "new" is not actually new at all.

It isn't even old.

It's ancient.

Chapter Two

Creating My Diet: Frankie Boy's Journey to Optimal Health

My journey to pursue optimal human health started on Google. I searched "what is the healthiest diet?" Literally. That was about seven years ago at a time when I was dealing with physical problems and living an unhealthy lifestyle.

But I only realized it was unhealthy in hindsight.

At the time, I thought I was doing everything right. I was following the classic nutritional playbook for weightlifting, something I had been practicing seriously for more than a half-decade. My focus was bodybuilding and gaining muscle. So, yeah, it turns out that I was the stereotypical New York Italian meathead way before I ever became a carnivore "meathead." Gym. Tan. Laundry. Chicken. Rice. Broccoli.

It took me a long time — and taking a step back to gain an outside perspective — to really understand that almost every aspect of bodybuilding culture is negative. From unrealistic expectations to rampant steroid use to gymrats killing their joints with marathon lifting sessions, none of it is actually healthy.

Despite building an enviable body and eating a diet approved by fitness influencers, nutritionists and doctors, I felt like shit. Things deteriorated further after I took Accutane, a prescription pharmaceutical, to fix my cystic acne. I was in my early 20s with a range of health problems. The worst was an inability to properly digest carbohydrates. All of a sudden, I had no energy despite eating pounds and pounds of grilled chicken, sweet potatoes, and brown rice every day.

Enough was enough. What I was doing wasn't working. Something had to change. This is what prompted my initial exploration into nutrition with that simple Google search.

I was open minded. I was willing to start at square one. I set off in search of health — not gains. With a little luck, and by finding some new knowledge that made me question everything I had been taught, I was able to forget conventional wisdom. That was the moment everything in my life turned for the better.

Indigenous Wisdom: Roots of the Ancestral Diet

Early on, I began to come across more and more information about the diets of indigenous groups and our hunter-gatherer ancestors.

I already had been following a Paleo Diet for awhile before discovering research into native diets, and this information was drastically different. Paleo, at the time, as practiced by most people, was mostly lean meats, vegetables, sweet potatoes, fruits, nuts, and seeds. This was billed as what people would have consumed before agriculture.

My friend told me to "eat the rainbow." I remember trying to eat at least a dozen different fruits and vegetables every single day on top of all the other recommended foods. On paper, according to modern standards, it was a perfect diet. But it wasn't working.

Then I started to learn just how incomplete — and simply wrong — a lot of this was. I was starting to learn about what our ancestors actually ate.

"How to Eat, Move, and be Healthy," by Paul Chek, was the first book that turned me on to studying indigenous diets. My mind was opened up by the early writings of Weston Price, a pioneering Canadian dentist who founded the National Dental Association and examined indigenous groups across the world in the early 1900s. I took a lot away from "The Fat of the Land," a book by Vilhjalmur Stefansson, an arctic explorer and Harvard-educated anthropologist who lived with indigenous Inuit Eskimos for years.

From these three men, and other sources I found along the way, I came away realizing one thing: Every group of indigenous people depended upon certain animal foods to survive.

Once I studied these foods, I learned that they have incredibly high amounts of vitamins. And the forms of these vitamins are very different from those found in plant foods. This instilled in me the idea that the presence of these nutrient-dense animal foods in the human diet is the most important factor for health, especially during developmental periods of life.

It became undeniable once I started eating like this. What really sold it was when I tasted these foods. I felt an almost-instant energy boost, especially when consuming liver and fish eggs.

Close to Home

This final factor is something that has always resonated with me for very personal reasons. Fixing my own health problems, having more energy, looking better, and generally improving my whole life were major motivations for my health journey. But my desire to learn more about nutrition also goes deeper.

I am a triplet, and my sister was unfortunately born mentally disabled. I had always known that triplets tend to have a harder time in infancy because it is difficult for one mother to nurse multiple newborns. Because of this, we were largely raised on soy formula that I was allergic to.

To make matters worse, my mother also had a botched cesarean procedure. She spent months in the hospital and nearly died. She underwent countless dialysis treatments before eventually receiving the double kidney transplant that kept her alive. Needless to say, fighting for her own life left my mother not only unable to provide all the nutritional needs of three newborns but staring down the barrel at a lifelong personal health struggle that she continues to battle with to this day.

I can never know exactly what circumstances led to my sister's condition and how much any nutritional deficiencies may have played a role. But I personally believe that dietary factors and stress on my mother may have contributed to my sister's developmental issues. In every newborn, there are specific bacteria that can only be obtained through natural childbirth and breastfeeding that helps cultivate a healthy microbiome.

This always weighed heavily on my mind when I thought about health. It is a big reason that learning more about the links between diet and human development became a passion.

In recent years, I have also applied the principles I've learned to help my sister lose a ton of weight. She is 4'11" and spent most of her life suffering with obesity. By transitioning to animal-based, carnivore eating — along with some calorie restriction early on — she has become much healthier and has much more energy. Physically, she is now skinny and in the best shape of her life. She will always face challenges. But she is now able to live a fuller, less-sedentary lifestyle, and what she eats is the biggest reason.

The Variety of Indigenous Diets

Due to my own family history, I was particularly struck by indigenous traditions surrounding pregnancy, breastfeeding, and infant development.

Weston Price wrote that the Massai, a semi-nomadic cattle-herding people in Kenya and Tanzania, would allot a ration of raw cow's blood for pregnant women, nursing mothers, and young children as long as it was available. The indigenous people of Fiji would gather certain shellfish to give to expectant mothers, and many coastal people would do the same thing with fish roe. Similar practices have been reported across the globe with different prized foods that we know to be incredibly nutrient dense — but that have been largely abandoned in modern U.S. culture.

Why have we gone against our own history? Why do we no longer eat like our grandparents — let alone our wise ancestors Why have convenience, processed crap, and unnaturally palatable foods become the foundation of the modern diet?

Looking back, indigenous people got the majority of their calories from animal foods. By some estimates, there are some groups that derived three-fourths of calories from animal sources (although two-thirds was likely closer to the norm). In pre-agricultural times, the rest of the hunter-gatherer diet came from wild plants, which were increasingly replaced by harvested grains within settled civilizations of the past few thousand years.

There were certain groups of people, particularly Inuit Eskimos and certain Plains Indians, who got drastically higher rates — even above 85% — of their calories from animal foods. That said, most native people did eat plant foods in some form.

Knowing this, why do I personally follow a carnivore diet that consists entirely of animal foods?

A few reasons. One is that ancestral indigenous groups mostly ate these plant foods out of necessity. Today, by contrast, I never have a problem finding more than enough animal foods to meet my energy needs. Two is that the modern plant foods that we have access to are far different from the ones our ancestors consumed.

Then there is inflammation. Removing all plant foods also allows for an elimination-style approach to understanding how different foods affect your body. And, from a calorie perspective, it also just tends to be easier and less expensive to purchase quality animal foods.

More than anything, my decision to eliminate plant food ties in to food quality — far and away the biggest factor in optimizing your health.

Food Quality Is King

Before we even consider the exact makeup of ancient diets, it is critical that we understand that the food these people were consuming was all of the highest quality. The animals were either wild game that truly lived naturally or livestock raised on pristine pasture. Today, even consumers who only eat organic usually fail to realize that food quality — whether it is fruits, vegetables, or animals — is directly linked to the quality of soil and the season of the year.

That gallon of pasteurized, homogenized, white, bland milk from the supermarket is miles away from the deep yellow, nutty, sweet, and delicious raw, grass-fed milk straight from the farm. And even today's farm-raised, grass-fed animals are, in the context of nutrient density, largely well below the standard of quality of those our ancestors ate. Because our soil, and thus the pasture our livestock eat, has become depleted of minerals and elements after decades of agricultural production.

You know how they say "you are what you eat?" Well, the same goes for a cow. And even the humanely raised, grass-fed cows of 2019 are eating grass that is much less nutritious than the livestock that were being raised during the height of the Roman Empire. And if the pasture they eat is less nutritious for them, eating them is less nutritious for us. Animals today are also slaughtered too young, not grazing for enough time in natural patterns.

It gets worse. Not only is today's milk missing the nutrient content it is supposed to have, modern pasteurization destroys the beneficial enzymes and bacteria that contribute to a healthy microbiome. Homogenization makes the fat globules more likely to cause gut issues due to the artificial particle size. Other modern production factors similarly make other foods oxidized and rancid, causing inflammation.

The same goes for plants. Forget the fact that the kale and broccoli we eat today didn't even exist in the past. Even compared to the vegetables that our great grandparents ate, the nutritional content of modern crops is dramatically lower.

This means that we need to work very hard to source the highest quality foods we can find.

This means purchasing grass-fed pastured beef over grain-fed meat, especially for fat and organs because that is where the animal stores its vitamins. It means selecting wild-caught fish over farm-raised salmon to optimize Omega-3 ratios and reduce pollution concerns. It means going to the farmer's market for pastured eggs since conventionally raised chickens are fed corn and soy that leave them full of undesirable Omega-6 fatty acids. It means striving to find raw dairy, if you tolerate it, to improve your nutrient intake and remove the negative effects associated with feedlot cattle. It means making sure shellfish is from the best available water source. In doing so, you remove as many inflammatory factors as possible, and optimize your consumption of vitamins, minerals, elements, and fatty acids.

It all sounds exhausting honestly, and, believe me, I know it can be. But devoting energy to sourcing high-quality food has become essential. It is unfortunate that we have reached this point. It is, however, the only real path to living better and feeling great.

My Diet, My Mission

All over New York and everywhere I travel, I see unhappy people. Fat. Sick. Depressed. Unhealthy. I see it in my mother, my father, and my sister. I used to see it in the mirror — even when I was living in the gym and convinced I was eating perfectly. Even now, I have to question what's going on with our national food supply and eating habits when I am the only healthy-looking person on the street.

It breaks my heart that so many of the problems of our modern life would have never occurred if we were living even in the recent past. There are many people on this planet suffering through desperate conditions. No, a better diet cannot fix everything and, yes, modern medicine and technologies have helped millions who would have died or suffered through much worse had they been born just a few centuries ago.

But millions of others can attribute some of their biggest issues to the processed, nutrient-devoid food of convenience that they eat today. It doesn't take much to change all that. They really can start living a better life if they start giving their bodies the basic vitamins, minerals, elements, and other things it needs. People have been doing it for tens of thousands of years. It just takes a little bit of knowledge, some level of commitment, and the realization that the standard American diet bears no resemblance to how human beings are meant to eat.

Helping these people — and you — is my goal. By providing the information, educating people on the importance of nutrients that can only be found in animal foods, and showing modern society the forgotten wisdom of our ancestors, your author Frankie Boy hopes that he can inspire many more people to wake up every day feeling great. With a little luck, you too might even look like a Roman statue forged in marble.

This is the reason why I started my YouTube channel. This is why I have published hundreds of videos over the past few years. This is why I am now writing a book that details my philosophy of nutrition and the core principles of the Ancestral Indigenous Diet. And this is why I hope you will come to understand just how important it is to obtain all the essential nutrients that were once a staple of every human diet.

I have already taken the long journey toward achieving my own optimal health.

Now, it's time for you to come along.

Chapter Three

The Fundamental Four: The Nutritional Foundation of the Ancestral Indigenous Diet

Our ancestors probably didn't think much about nutrition. They acted on instinct, living naturally in the sun, eating wild foods, and sleeping under the stars. But there are signs that they understood that eating certain things were beneficial even if they didn't know the difference between Omega-3 and Omega-6 fats or why the animal form of Vitamin A (retinol) is more bioavailable and beneficial to humans than the plant form (beta-carotene).

They praised organ meats like liver and kidneys, and they knew — whether instinctively or through generations of passed-on wisdom — to eat bone marrow. Yes, they probably spent most of their time trying to obtain calories and they definitely didn't understand the science behind the fact that wild animals store the critical vitamins we need in their organs, fat stores, and marrow. But nature and learned knowledge had a way of compelling them to consume the nutrients that they needed most.

"Hunting man is a connoisseur of fats and has a definite sequence of preferences in the different fats according to their origination in different parts of the body," wrote adventurer Vilhjalmur Stefansson about the Inuit preferences for caribou in his landmark 1956 book *The Fat of the Land*. "The marrows are best, and range in excellence from the hip and shoulder joints down — the farther down, the better … The ratings in descending order are: the fat from behind the eye, the kidney fat, the fat on the brisket near the bone, the fat of the ribs, and other parts where it is mixed with the lean. Last comes the back fat."

When seeking fat and organs, these people might not have known that Vitamin A is important for eye health. But many did understand that consuming eyeballs — a food high in Vitamin A — would fix eye problems. They also knew what foods to eat during various stages of development, something we know was practiced by various groups. They would feed certain items to nursing mothers, couples trying to conceive, people dealing with illness, and older members of the community.

We see similar practices — even among groups still living apart from modern society today — when it comes to medicine and hydration. Indigenous groups living deep in the Amazon cannot tell you about the biochemistry and other processes that regulate immune system responses. But they know exactly what type of tree bark may help treat hernia and what vines they can cut down to acquire a safe source of drinking water.

Their understanding of the natural world around them, and especially their diet, was somewhat mechanistic in this sense. Over thousands of years and hundreds of generations, collective wisdom was learned and passed down. This practical knowledge became essential to their health and survival. It's a shame that it has been lost in just a few decades.

This was their "conventional wisdom." But it has somehow mostly been lost to time, replaced by decades of rapid change that has provided some invaluable scientific insight — especially about bacteria and pathogens — but has also largely been warped by an underlying drive to feed as many people as possible, as cheaply as possible.

But optimal human health for the individual fell by the wayside. From the top, everything about discussion moved toward the goal of preventing acute nutrient deficiencies among a population of 330 million people. And all of the advice is wrapped up in the underlying biased view that mass production and transportation of food is necessary. Guidelines from the FDA only consider if preservatives and additives are actually toxic rather than starting from a viewpoint that none of this should be in our food!

Massive corporations came to dominate the food supply. Their goal was not to raise animals that provide people with the best nutrition. They wanted to raise animals as cheaply as possible. This meant keeping cows indoors on relatively small feedlots and force-feeding them the cheapest feed available. They were given corn and soy that were drenched with agrochemicals that would help these crops grow faster. Then they pumped the cows with steroids and hormones to get even more meat per cow. And to keep the animals from catching diseases and dying before slaughter due to this horrific lifestyle, they had to shoot them full of antibiotics.

The same thing was happening for plant foods. The focus was always on maximizing yield and engineering drought- and blight-resistant crops. There were good intentions — helping society avoid the famines of the past that killed so many people. This was great! But those noble goals would be overtaken by corporate profit goals, and the nutrient content of plants would plummet over the decades.

Why? The answer is always money.

The Dorito Effect, a 2015 book by author Mark Schatzker, details just how drastically that modern farming practices and crop engineering has taken away from plant foods in something the scientists that conducted the research have called "The Dilution Effect." The following represent just a few of the many changes highlighted. "1950s kale had twice as much riboflavin (Vitamin B2) as modern kale. 1950s cauliflower had twice as much thiamine (Vitamin B1). And 1950s asparagus had almost three times as much ascorbic acid (Vitamin C) … It was as though modern produce had been nutritionally dumbed down."

The government's role in all of this is also not motivated by improving the health of individuals. They merely evaluate all the unnatural parts of the process and decide whether this chemical, that hormone, or some other antibiotic will cause serious damage to the consumer.

They do not ever say the obvious: None of this should be in our food! And they don't warn people that, beyond all the negative substances, the end product is meat that is much lower in the nutrients we need to live in optimal health.

The decline of food quality is the biggest factor in the decline of our health, as we will discuss much more in future chapters. For now, the key message to remember from this brief history is this: We have abandoned everything we learned over the past hundred thousand years. And while it may have helped to provide sustenance to billions of people more efficiently, it is now destroying our individual health.

Eating Our Way to an Early Grave

In much of the United States, at least among almost everyone reading this book, there is no longer a need to worry about caloric scarcity. The problem is the opposite. Overconsumption is now the norm because we have too much access to unnaturally palatable food.

But even as people eat more and more, they get less and less of what they actually need. Past humans went days — sometimes weeks — without food at times. We can't go three hours without a snack.

Nobody thinks that candy and potato chips have any nutritional value, but people really do believe that brown rice, fruit, and store-bought yogurt give them everything they need. People even think in very simple terms — saying "this is healthy" as they eat a smoothie full of sugar but no nutrients to speak of — and then go about their day without realizing they are lacking many of the key building blocks of actual health.

What is missing? Depending upon what they eat, it may be many things. But there are a few absolutely essential components that humans need. These are the vitamins, and one fatty acid, that you need to really prioritize and understand if you are going to reach your optimal health. Without question, there are more things that you must obtain to hit this goal. But by prioritizing these three vitamins, and one fatty acid, the rest will all mostly fall into place naturally.

This is our scientific answer; we know these nutrients are important for our health. The logical answer ties into ancestral diets, these animal nutrients were present across all native indigenous groups.

To make it easier and take some of the confusion out of eating, this book starts with these, "The Fundamental Four," that will make up the foundation of nutrient density. This doesn't mean the others (which we will discuss in the following chapter) are necessarily less important. But these four are often lacking and poorly understood.

If you start here, get back to basics, and start to obtain each of these foundational nutrients, you will quickly be on your way to eating — and feeling — better.

The Keys of Nutrient Density

Before getting into the specific vitamins and fat that we need, it's important to understand the core philosophy behind this diet. The goal of the Ancestral Indigenous Diet is to eat the most nutritionally dense foods possible while completely avoiding anything that may be detrimental (by causing inflammation, introducing anti-nutrients, harming our gut, or generally disrupting the natural mechanisms within our bodies).

This requires eating high-quality animal foods, and the good news is that we can obtain all the nutrients we need without even consuming a ton of calories. By eating the right items (like liver, certain seafood, and the correct cheese), we will have everything we need.

But beyond nutrients, we of course also need enough calories to fuel our bodies to stay alive as well as enough protein to rebuild cells, tissues, and muscles. After we hit our nutritional goals, those two areas become the priority.

The other key goal when eating will be to eliminate inflammation. We will cover that deeper in a later chapter — but this is one of the key reasons that plant foods are not just unnecessary but potentially harmful. We will also dig deeper into why I don't consume plant foods later in the book.

But before we really detail what we should eat, we need to understand the why.

Why are different nutrients so important? Which nutrients should you focus on when designing your diet? What are the common deficiencies and how do you avoid missing out on the things your body needs most?

We will begin to explore all of that right now. But, at the same time, this isn't a biology textbook. My goal in the next two chapters is to provide an overview of the primary vitamins and nutrients that I believe should be nutritional foundation of your diet and the key reasons that you need to be obtaining them. I want to give you the practical information that will help you recognize why you need these nutrients. I do not want to drone on with so much science and so many research studies that you forget it all by tomorrow.

This is why I will focus on mechanisms within the body and continue to express how important it was for our indigenous ancestors to consume these nutrients. Hopefully, by taking this approach, you can come to understand why I place such a priority on these specific nutrients in my diet.

Vitamin A

If you look at a typical nutrition resource online, it will tell you that Vitamin A is important for maintaining healthy teeth, bones, soft tissue, mucous membranes, and skin. It will note Vitamin

A's role in eye health and tell you that its scientific names (retinol, retinal, and retinoic acid) are related to its role in producing pigments in the retina of the eye. You might learn that Vitamin A deficiency can lead to blindness.

While these factors are certainly important, there is much more to know. Along with the other fat-soluble vitamins we will discuss, Vitamin A is critical to cell differentiation and gene expression — the process by which essentially every cell is made in the body.

Because this process is the foundation of everything, the importance of these vitamins is understated in human biology. Most people will go their whole lives without even understanding what this is or how our diet can impact these functions.

In the simplest terms, gene expression turns on and off genes to regulate what cells your body needs, and cell differentiation is the act of those cells becoming specialized cells (such as white blood cells or a stem cell). Genes are what determine all of the characteristics of our bodies that regulate function.

The fact that most diets are lacking in the nutrients key to such basic cell function can likely explain the poor health of most people. All of these fat-soluble vitamins are tied together in complex metabolic chains involving other vitamins, minerals, elements, fatty acids, and pretty much anything that enters your body.

So, while Vitamin A is not unique in its effect on this process, it does have a significant role to play. In the context of gene expression, retinoic acid in fact regulates hundreds of genes in the body, including stem cell differentiation (meaning the production of stem cells), and germ cell differentiation in embryonic development. Overall, it plays a role in the regulation of more than 500 genes!

And most people are not consuming nearly enough Vitamin A to make sure all of these vital processes are regulated properly. But they think they are — due to an entirely different form of poor regulation: This time from the U.S. government.

Through the Institute of Medicine (IOM), the established Recommended Dietary Allowances (RDA) and Dietary Reference Intakes (DRI) allow the beta-carotene from plant foods to be labeled as Vitamin A (in the form of retinol activity equivalents, or RAE). But this substance, also known as "Provitamin A," is not what our body actually needs.

These carotenoids need to be converted by the body into the usable retinal form (or "preformed Vitamin A"), and the conversion rates can vary significantly by person. In fact, many people only convert beta-carotene in very small amounts. And this process can be further impaired in various ways, including certain gene differences between people and compounds in plant foods that inhibit certain enzymes involved in conversion.

In short, (1) the animal form of Vitamin A is the most bioavailable for our bodies, and (2) some of us can only get it in high amounts from a few specific sources (namely liver and high-quality egg yolks). If you are eating carrots and kale every day and thinking all those carotenoids are doing the job, you may be sorely mistaken.

All this also brings up another important point to understand about the RDAs: They were created to help prevent deficiencies in 97.5% of the population — not to promote optimal health. Besides that, they have been updated only once (in 2016) since being established in 1968.

Why exactly are we taking advice from a government body that updates its information every 50 years? And should we be merely trying to prevent deficiencies or actually optimize our intake?

Really, the importance of Vitamin A cannot be overstated. And as much as all of the fat-soluble vitamins are essential, starting to consume foods high in Vitamin A is one way that many people can create a noticeable difference in their health almost immediately.

Vitamin A: Sources & Preparation

Of all the so-called "superfoods" touted by "experts" and magazine articles, there may be nothing better to consume than liver. Whether it's from cow, lamb, chicken, duck, other birds, cod, or other fish, liver is the only food source in nature that is truly high in Vitamin A.

That being said, it's safe to say that not every person in every tribe was able to get enough liver to eat. Each animal only has one, and it isn't that large relative to muscle meat, fat, and even other organs. But even small ocean fish, shellfish, and insects either have small stores of Vitamin A in their livers or are just much higher in Vitamin A than the foods we eat now. So our ancestors were able to get by even when the big-game hunting wasn't going so well.

This was fine because, in general, people don't even need all that much. Even 100 grams of liver a week is probably sufficient depending upon body size. That said, consumption should be prioritized early on. Eating more is likely a good idea because most people living on a Standard American Diet will have deficiencies. And this applies not just to Vitamin A but for most of the fundamental nutrients. Whereas indigenous people in the past were getting adequate levels starting in the womb, you are going to have to make up for some lost time in the beginning phase.

In our modern days, cod liver supplements are an option for people who don't like liver or have a hard time sourcing it locally. And this isn't just a modern diet fad like most supplements you find online or from big retailers. Your grandparents can all likely tell you about the awful taste when they were force-fed spoonfuls as a kid. Fortunately, today's versions have a better flavor, but people have been relying on fish liver oil for a long, long time.

"Scandanavian fishermen often have a belief in the nearly magical value of cod or halibut liver oil, and some of them will toss off, most likely in the morning, the equivalent of a wineglassful," wrote Stefansson in *The Fat of the Land*.

Canned cod liver is generally easier to find — and more approachable in terms of taste, as are poultry liver (chicken, duck, goose) or baby animal livers (like veal and lamb). Beef, goat, and pig liver, by comparison, are all much stronger tasting and some find them to simply be unpalatable. One note, however: Food quality ties in directly to flavor. Grass-fed, naturally raised ruminant liver, even coming from an older animal, will taste significantly better than conventionally raised beef liver.

Other benefits from cod liver (and other fish livers) are their large amounts of Omega-3 fatty acids and Iodine, while poultry livers tend to have higher amounts of Vitamin K2. And as with beef, the taste is improved when the animal lived a natural life on the farm — not to mention the overall nutrient profile of liver. Freshly slaughtered meat is also far more mild in taste. So if you get liver that hasn't been sitting in a store freezer for months, it will be less disagreeable even to people who don't like the flavor. There is also natural variation in all cases. Beef liver, for example, is higher in B Vitamins, whereas goose liver is higher in Vitamin K2 and duck liver has a lot of iron.

While it does pay to find a way to consume some form of liver, those who simply cannot choke anything down can get (much) smaller amounts from eggs or certain dairy. But the chickens must be truly free-range. And the milk must be non-pasteurized and come from grass-fed cows. Otherwise, the Vitamin A content is very hard to know and will likely be negligible.

A store-bought carton of milk is left with no natural Vitamin A. But manufacturers do often add synthetic Vitamin A in the form of retinyl palmitate — which can be harmful to the human liver. This is just one more reason to stay away from conventional dairy.

Because high-quality versions of these foods are often hard to source dependably, liver is always the best way to go. Especially at the beginning as you make up for your (likely) past deficiency. In time, as you replenish Vitamin A stores, you may do OK getting by just on eggs, raw dairy, and other grass-fed animal fat.

In any case, effort into food sourcing and preparation is important. Canned cod liver and various pâtés are available or can even be made at home. It's as simple as sautéing some liver, and blending it up with some raw cream, raw butter, and raw honey. This is super high nutrient, tasty, and approachable. It's like liver ice cream. Dip some slices of raw parmesan cheese in it (or some type of a cracker that is healthier if you must).

You can also of course just sauté or grill liver all by itself. It can be very bitter and astringent from low quality, conventionally raised animals. Buying grass-fed, especially younger animals will alleviate this. If you only have access to low-quality liver, soaking it for 24 hours in milk (or water or anything you can think of really), is a good option.

I prefer to dry out the surface after marinating by leaving it on a rack in the fridge overnight, and then pan searing it the next day in butter. Eating it this way with liberal salt and pepper, or along with bites of cheese or even topped with some hot sauce, can make it easy to consume 100 grams or so a few times a week, which is plenty to get the Vitamin A you need.

I've also put liver on a wood fire, and this is an OK option but not really my favorite. Depending on how strict you are and what your dietary goals are you can also use various types of flour to bread it and fry it, although I don't think it's really necessary if you marinate the liver and dry it out properly. The Eskimos preferred to boil liver, and some tribes ate it raw.

Really, I've tried everything — even swallowing down raw liver in the past. So if you are all for obtaining your nutrition just by swallowing the liver, you can. It's just that there are more enjoyable ways.

Omega-3 Fatty Acids

As already mentioned, the other fat-soluble vitamins are crucial. But before moving on to those, I want to talk about another component of a healthy diet that has many people confused: Omega-3 fatty acids.

By now, everybody knows that they are important. Perhaps no supplement has gotten more marketing in the past decade than fish oil and its role in providing us with the Omega-3s we need. But even with all the recommendations, people remain misguided about why they are so critical to consume

First off, many of these Omega fatty acids must be obtained through the diet, but it goes far beyond simply popping a few pills. Because on top of just getting an allotted amount of milligrams per day, you need to properly balance your Omega-3 levels with the other fats you consume, namely the Omega-6s that are severely over-consumed on the standard American diet.

While I don't want to overcomplicate this, there is some more granular information that you do need to know to get this all right. For starters, there are actually three different types of Omega 3s: EPA (eicosapentaenoic acid), DHA (docosahexaenoic acid), and ALA (alpha-linolenic acid).

EPA and DHA — the two types found only in animal foods — are our bread and butter. That is what you need to focus on acquiring every day. These fatty acids primarily help regulate cellular inflammation (EPA) and maintain optimal brain health, nerve cell structure, and nerve cell function (DHA). While EPA produces beneficial chemicals called eicosanoids that are involved in anti-inflammatory processes, we absolutely must always prioritize DHA because it is a requirement for the brain, which uses these acids at a rate of around 4.6 mg per day. The role of DHA is essential in early human development and its levels in breast milk can vary from 0.06% to 1.4% — a 20-fold variance!

For one real-world example, we may be able to look at the vascular properties of the indigenous Inuit "Eskimos" in northern Canada. Likely due to their high DHA and EPA consumption, as chronicled by Weston Price in the early 1900s, their blood clotted much slower, at around nine minutes, than the average of four minutes for people living in the United States. This is due to platelet adhesiveness as well as concentration of fibrinogen in the blood.

And when their blood is flowing that smoothly, no wonder they didn't have any heart disease to speak of!

The third type, ALA, is Omega-3 form predominantly found in plant foods, especially seed oils (generally branded as "vegetable oils") like canola, soybean, corn, safflower, and palm oils. Once consumed, ALA can be stored in adipose tissue and used for energy production.

There is a widespread belief that getting the animal forms of Omega-3s directly is unnecessary because the body can convert ALA into EPA and DHA. But this is more myth than science in a practical sense. The conversion of ALA to EPA is minimal, generally at less than 5%, and ALA consumption has not been shown to raise blood levels of DHA in any studies.

In a more theoretical sense, conversion rates can likely be greater. But this doesn't happen efficiently in the presence of high Omega-6 levels — which are nearly universal in the modern U.S. diet (especially among vegetarians and vegans who often lack EPA and DHA).

Without turning this into a science textbook, this is because Omega-6 fatty acids compete for the Delta 6 Desaturase enzyme for conversion at multiple stages of its metabolism to DHA. And when almost everyone consumes a high-Omega-6 diet, this process is significantly impaired.

Along similar lines, many indigenous groups are believed to have been completely free from heart disease, and one proposed factor in this is the absence of seed oils and other highly processed modern food.

Lastly, it must be noted that high Omega-6 levels can cause mitochondrial cell death and are generally a driving factor for many diseases. Linoleic acid, a commonly consumed Omega-6 fatty acid, can trigger necrotic cell death when obtained in abnormal amounts, whereas conjugated linoleic acid (an Omega-6 found in animal foods) has almost the reverse effect.

What this and the rest of the information tells us is that we need to maintain the right balance between Omega-6s and Omega-3s — a ratio that has gotten further and further out of whack in recent decades.

In ancestral times, this ratio was probably right around 1 to 1 whereas it has now gone to more than 15 to 1, or even higher, according to a study from the [Center for Genetics, Nutrition, and Health](#) in Washington. "Western diets are deficient in Omega-3 fatty acids and have excessive amounts of Omega-6 fatty acids compared with the diet on which human beings evolved and their genetic patterns were established," stated a 2002 paper by Dr. Artemis Simopoulos, the center's founder.

More and more evidence is now showing that the runaway levels of Omega-6s — and the resulting inflammation they cause — in the modern diet is among the leading causes of our nation's health crisis, and their presence is largely looked as an intractable part of our entire way of eating. Because of this, Omega-3s are widely seen as a mere supplement that will help lessen the damage much the same way we are told to consume blueberries and wine for their antioxidant properties.

Essentially, people have been conned into thinking they can simply pop a fish oil pill each day and protect their heart from all the damage being done by the seed oils (and sugar) they stuff down their throats every day.

The market has taken advantage of this ignorance. It now pumps out billions of low-quality fish oil supplements filled with additives. So even if taking a small serving per day could do anything for you, it won't help if you're taking mass-produced pills that ignore the vital DHA and EPA to instead just pump you full of less-useful ALA. (These mass-market, low-quality pills are also often highly oxidized.)

DHA and Omega-3s must become a staple — not a supplement. Filling your diet with Omega-3s is critical because, as noted, both DHA and EPA are essential to core bodily functions. The goal is not to hit some small milligram marker that your doctor recommends. What you must do is get the ratio of Omega-3s to Omega-6s back in line with the natural eating that our ancestors practiced for the last hundred thousand years.

This requires doing some homework and understanding the different ratios in different foods. This is the reason why, beyond pesticides and dirty practices, that wild-caught salmon is so much more beneficial to your health. Because pollution in oceans can be very bad near the coast, farmed fish are honestly one of the most toxic foods to consume.

From a nutrient standpoint, yes, farm-raised Atlantic salmon does have more overall fat — and even more Omega-3s — than wild-caught sockeye salmon. But it is also chocked full of Omega-6s. Meanwhile, sockeye and other wild-caught varieties have almost no Omega-6s. So it doesn't matter that their overall Omega-3 content is also less. The nutrient profile is just so much better.

By eating sockeye, you improve your body's ratios. And while we will detail this all in more detail later, this is the same reason that eating conventionally raised chicken and pork is doing you no favors. Wild fowl and feral hogs do have good Omega ratios that are excellent for human consumption. But because the feedlot-raised varieties of these animals eat soy and corn instead of their natural foraging diet (which may include acorns and insects), their fat stores become laden with the same Omega-6s we are trying to avoid. These animals become what they eat just like you do.

Fixing your Omega ratio requires two practical steps: Increasing your Omega-3s (in the form of DHA and EPA) and cutting out the Omega-6s. That isn't something you can do with a pill or even by ordering a farm-raised salmon filet once a week. It takes a concerted effort.

Ultimately, fixing Omega ratios is something that will happen inherently over time when seed oils are removed and higher-quality foods start to make up the majority of your diet. But fish helps, and high-quality fish oils will speed up that process. This is key because an imbalanced ratio of Omega-3 to Omega-6 can increase oxidative stress — a driving factor for most diseases.

Omega-3: Sources & Preparation

There are two reasons that we need to focus on acquiring DHA, more so than EPA and ALA. First, the others are not nearly as important when it comes to human metabolism. And, secondly, EPA inherently comes alongside high-DHA foods in most cases. This is good news that simplifies everything: If you eat foods loaded in DHA, you will be good to go.

How do we do that? Seafood — and lots of it. The fattier the fish, the better (with wild-caught salmon being the most popular). Fish eggs (look for salmon roe) are even higher in DHA on a per-calorie basis and this makes them among the leading actual "superfoods" out there. Normal chicken eggs are probably the most approachable source of DHA, but they also have a high Omega-6 content due to grain feeding. So much like wild-caught vs. farm-raised fish, they are only a high-level option if they are truly free-range.

One other fantastic option is consuming animal brains, which are very high in DHA. Like fish eggs, their DHA is in the phospholipid form, which is said to be more available to our own brains. I eat them quite often, but most people understandably aren't going to go to such great lengths for their diet. But pan-seared lamb or veal brains are definitely worth a try — if you can find them and handle it.

When it comes to preparation, some people believe that fish is very tricky to cook. And it can be without any experience. But even novice cooks usually quickly learn that simply baking a salmon filet in an oven for 15 minutes with salt, pepper, and butter can be a delicious meal. Even better is sautéing a filet skin-down with a little bit of oil in a pan. It might take a few tries, but you will soon learn that you can cook it as rare or as well done as you like and come away with wonderfully crispy skin and the translucent pink flesh that chefs across the world would envy.

For ease and the best DHA density per calorie, I personally enjoy fish eggs as often as I can find them. While actual caviar is prohibitively expensive, salmon roe (or other types of roe) is often available from local fish purveyors in cities or Asian markets. All you need is a few tablespoons in a day a couple of times a week to get the DHA you need (when combined with a wider diet of other high-quality animal foods).

Sashimi is another favorite of mine, although it can get expensive eating it out and is a bit tedious to prepare yourself. Canned fish can work as well and things like sardines and anchovies are great for anyone on a budget.

Vitamin K2

Next on our list is a nutrient that most people overlook altogether when thinking about their health: Vitamin K2. This vitamin, in the form of MK7, is thought to play a role in skeletal health.

But its sister version, MK4, is far more important and can be converted to any other forms we need. Animal foods predominantly contain MK4, which also plays a key role in preventing calcium buildup in organs and tissues, including arteries.

In addition to these forms, there is Vitamin K1, which is commonly found in plant foods and cannot be efficiently converted to vitamin k2 in animal foods. Then there are a few other forms (MK8, MK9, MK10, and MK11) that each occur in different animal foods. But Vitamin K2 is arguably the most important of the group and, unfortunately, it's also the most difficult vitamin to obtain in our diets.

Another factor that makes Vitamin K2 so important is that it activates MGP (Matrix Gla Protein), which allows calcium to be properly transported in the body. And outside of vascular health, the series of "menaquinones" known collectively as Vitamin K2 are linked to exercise performance, sexual health, reducing insulin sensitivity, and, some studies show, protecting us from cancer.

This all sounds important. But what makes K2 more important than some of the other vitamins? Well, in general, it isn't that it is necessarily *more* important. It's just that many people don't get nearly enough of it. And this is easily fixable because it's largely due to them not placing any priority on Vitamin K2 and avoiding the few good sources that exist.

Unlike the B Vitamins that most people just accumulate by accident in their diet, you need to seek out Vitamin K2, largely in the form of fermented foods or high-quality eggs. All high-quality animal foods do contain small amounts of Vitamin K2. Liver and eggs are decent sources as well. But fermented foods like cheese are the key.

You also must make sure your gut health stays optimal so that the bacteria living there can continue producing at least some of what we need. Yes, the bugs living inside your intestines do some of the work for you here as long as you're not destroying your bowels with a bad diet and antibiotics.

"Little is known about the absorption and transport of Vitamin K produced by gut bacteria, but research indicates that substantial quantities ... are present in the large bowel," according to the National Institute of Health (NIH). "Although the amount of vitamin K that the body obtains in this manner is unclear, experts believe that these menaquinones satisfy at least some of the body's requirement for Vitamin K."

Vitamin K2: Sources & Preparation

Vitamin K2, like Vitamin A, is contained in many animal foods to some degree depending on the quality of the pasture. This is because chlorophyll in the grass converts into Vitamin K2 in the tissue of the animal. And this initial amount will then increase through fermentation.

As far as higher-volume sources, eggs are really the only food containing any significant amount of Vitamin K2 that you would cook. And, as with DHA, you are going to have much better results in this department by going with truly free-range eggs laid by birds that eat their natural diet outdoors.

The other good source comes in the form of fermented foods. This is because Vitamin K2 will develop more and more as the items age because, as they do in your gut, bacteria play a role in producing this essential vitamin.

Cheese is the obvious choice. But you won't be obtaining this nutrient from the bulk of the "cheese" you find in a supermarket. You need to be looking for grass-fed "raw" cheese (meaning that it was made from unpasteurized milk).

Various types from Europe tend to fit the bill. Some good choices are Parmigiano-Reggiano from Italy, the gruyere-like variety L'Étivaz from Switzerland, and Bleu d'Auvergne, among other famous blue cheeses from France. As a rule, if a cheese has received a formal designation of protection from its local jurisdiction, it means it is made the traditional way and will retain much of its natural nutrient content. Overall, cheese from Switzerland is probably the best, followed by France and Spain. Nation of origin doesn't guarantee quality, but these are usually better on average and each has specific cheeses that are always made in a more traditional, nutritious way.

In the United States, you will have the best luck at local farms that sell raw cheese or aged types (that can legally be made from unpasteurized dairy) in specialty stores (or even Whole Foods these days). Cheeses made from goat and sheep's milk also tend to be grass-fed more often than those coming from cow's milk because these animals generally live outside, at least for most of their lives, rather than in a feedlot prison.

Though the number of sources is somewhat limited for Vitamin K2, the good news is that it's all relatively palatable and easy to consume. All you need is good, aged cheeses and fermented meats. And as mentioned, keeping a healthy intestine will help out as well.

Vitamin D3

The last of the four fundamental nutrients discussed here is Vitamin D3. Like Vitamin A, it is a precursor to cell differentiation and gene expression for hundreds of genes. This means that it's importance often flies under the radar, with most resources only noting its role in calcium metabolism.

Given its association with hormones that signal absorption and release of calcium, it is definitely important for bone homeostasis. And through decades of Got Milk and It Does a Body Good advertisements, you have certainly heard about milk being fortified with Vitamin D to promote skeletal health (after most of the actual nutrients are killed through pasteurization).

But, as we can see in other key areas, this is only part of the story. Vitamin D3 is required for the production of many hormones and having low levels can be associated with many common human diseases. It has even been shown to be effective in cancer therapy. Doctors even seem to be catching on. They are conducting more tests and routinely recommending patients start supplementing. Even if their aim is usually to prevent bone degradation, the more widespread awareness of Vitamin D's importance has been a good development.

Still, there are two main issues that prevent many people from obtaining adequate levels. The first is the biggest reason: Everyone is scared of the sun. Humans have always gotten the bulk of their Vitamin D3 simply by living and spending a lot of time outdoors. Our bodies contain a "zoosterol" substance called 7-Dehydrocholesterol that can be photochemically converted to Vitamin D3 in the presence of UV light.

Throughout history, we used to be in the sun most of the day. Our "jobs" were essentially procuring food, and the only way to procure food was to hunt or harvest crops outside.

Getting enough UV light was definitely never a problem for anyone living near the equator. But far northern and southern latitudes may have had lower UV indexes for the majority of the year, meaning people native to these areas would have had to consume more Vitamin D3 from food sources.

That brings us to the second problem that modern people have when it comes to reaching adequate levels: food quality. Thousands of years ago, even people living in areas like Russia could get enough Vitamin D3 from food. This is because, just like humans, other animals convert UV sunlight into Vitamin D3. Wild game, fish, and even livestock before the last few decades would spend all day outside and accumulate a substantial amount. All humans need to do was eat these animals in a large enough quantity — which they were already doing just to get calories for energy — and they would be all set.

Even when looking at more modern Russian indigenous groups, their Vitamin D3 levels can range from around 40 ng/ml to 67 ng/ml (nanograms/milliliter) — triple the amount that most people have today. That 40 ng/ml mark is a key threshold because this is when your body will have more than enough for all current needs and start storing Vitamin D3 for the winter.

Any lower than that and you are essentially running on empty anytime the sun rays are sparse. Depending who you ask, anywhere from 40 ng/ml to 80 ng/ml has been deemed healthy. The National Institute of Health considers 12 ng/ml or less as a "deficiency." But it notes that even between 12 ng/ml and 20 ng/ml is "generally considered inadequate for bone and overall health in healthy individuals."

With all that said, what does this really mean? While screening for Vitamin D3 levels is a good idea, these blood levels aren't something you will be tracking regularly. And, unfortunately, we have another RDA-related problem here.

The RDA recommendation of 600 IU (international units) per day for people 70 years old or younger is actually based on a statistical fallacy. Shockingly, the real Vitamin D3 RDA should always have been at least 10 times that figure — something that more and more scientists are coming to sound the alarm about.

Specifically, studies from UC San Diego and Creighton University in 2015 led to the publication of a letter in the journal *Nutrients* that advocated for a correction. "We call for the IOM and all public health authorities concerned with transmitting accurate nutritional information to the public to designate, as the RDA, a value of approximately 7000 IU per day from all sources," wrote Dr. Robert Heaney of Creighton University.

One hell of a mistake, huh? Another study in Nutrients ("A Statistical Error in the Estimation of the Recommended Dietary Allowance for Vitamin D") found that the correct calculation may even be as high as 8,895 IU per day. But many have understood this error for a long time, based upon the knowledge that the body can produce over 40,000 IU per day. Finally, the nutrition world is starting to come around now.

In a sad way, this is a great metaphor for all areas of our modern diet. After decades of thinking and moving in the wrong direction, some people are finally starting to recognize just how out of whack everything is.

Vitamin D3: Sources & Preparation

Knowing these numbers is helpful. But only to a point for the average person. Whether our target is 60 ng/ml or 7,000(+) IU/day, how do we get this much Vitamin D3?

Getting some sun is the best way to go and then you can also rely on high-quality food sources, supplements, or even tanning beds. People worry about skin cancer now more than ever, and there is reason to be cautious. But especially if the rest of your nutrition is spot on — and you are getting enough Vitamin A, which works somewhat in concert with Vitamin D3 — you are probably worrying more than you need to.

Always consult with your physician, but in most cases, getting more sun will usually do more good than harm even when you factor in the level of potential risk. The amount of sun exposure you want also depends upon various factors. You need to understand the UV index at different geographies and different times of year.

During the winter, even in a relatively sunny place like Los Angeles, for example, you wouldn't get nearly as much Vitamin D3 from the sun because of the tilt of the earth. Without getting too scientific, sunlight is composed of two types of UV light, called UVB and UVA rays. In the summer in most areas, this is actually around 95% UVA and 5% UVB during much of the day. And Vitamin D3 conversion is the product of UVB rays. So sunbathing from 8 am to 10 am might not actually do you that much good.

During the "peak UV" hours from around 11 am to 1 pm, however, the UVB percentage may be as high as 20%. So, while you want to be careful and understand how your individual skin reacts to a clear day at peak UV, you can get a lot more bang for your buck in a shorter duration of exposure midday. (And as noted, this depends significantly on your latitude. People in Maine, Florida, and Ecuador all experience very different UVB concentrations at different times of the year and different times of day.)

Vitamin D3 conversion can also vary depending upon skin color. If you are outside at peak UV during warmer months, the amount of absorption may be drastically different between people with pale white skin, olive skin, brown skin, and black skin. Our ancestors would have adapted to the sun slowly during the course of the spring, so when the scorching summer heat came, their skin was ready for it.

There are also diminishing returns on sun exposure — for any person in any location — related to how often you are outside as well as how your skin progressively tans. As a rule, it is usually better to be outside in the sun for one hour per day in peak UV than it is to be outside seven hours once per week. Your skin can only absorb so much per day, so it is ideal to spread it out frequently. This will also prevent you from overdoing it and risking sunburn.

For people living in Minneapolis in January — and, really, just anyone at any time who can't get outside midday very often — tanning beds are an alternative. The one thing to watch out for, however, is the UVA/UVB ratio. Many tanning beds fall in line with the sun in regard to this ratio but, because both tan your skin equally well, some have very low UVB levels. This can be as low as 1% — or less. So be sure to ask or look up the model of the tanning bed to make sure it will provide you with the necessary UVB rays that are essential to Vitamin D3 production. (Tanning beds also have electromagnetic field, EMF, concerns that should be understood before risking this option.)

As with our Russian and Norwegian ancestors, food is also a good source of Vitamin D3 for people today. The only problem is that feedlot cows and conventionally raised chicken generally spend much of their life inside. So, in addition to all the other aforementioned problems that this creates nutritionally, they also don't contain the natural levels of Vitamin D3 of wild game or grass-fed, free-grazing beef. The same goes for conventional dairy and eggs, although these are sometimes fortified with Vitamin D3 (although the other nutritional downsides make them not worth consuming ultimately).

For that reason, for most people, fatty fish like mackerel, herring, sardines, and anchovies are the best easily accessible and affordable sources. Fish roe is also great. Wild-caught is always best for all seafood, although farmed fish likely contains more nutrients than farmed land animals.

Ultimately, if you're wondering whether an animal source will be high or low in Vitamin D3, ask yourself this: Did it live in the sun for most of its life? If the answer is "no," its meat, fat, and byproducts won't contain much Vitamin D3. Make sense?

Another thing to consider is supplementation. This can be useful for anyone and particularly so for the Minneapolis college student in January who can't afford grass-fed beef or tanning beds. Vitamin D3 supplements are relatively cheap, although you want to find a well-regarded brand.

If you do go with drops or pills, be sure to keep this in mind: Vitamin D3 in supplement form is metabolized differently than it is from the sun. It's absorbed much faster. So certain precautions should be made. Instead of taking a large amount of Vitamin D3 drops or pills all at once, it is ideal to spread it out over the course of the day. (Many people find it better to take earlier in the day the better, as it can sometimes cause sleeping issues if taken too late at night.)

Lastly there is one final consideration: Vitamin D3 also goes hand in hand with Vitamin K2, which binds to calcium and transports it into and out of various tissues. In nature, we would likely not have obtained Vitamin D3 without Vitamin K2. Chances are, if we were in the sun for long periods of time, we were eating quality animal foods that contain Vitamin K2. In modern times, when supplementation is popular, this is something you need to keep in mind (although following the Ancestral Indigenous Diet means you will always be prioritizing both).

In the context of fixing past deficiencies, Vitamin D3 can be loaded at the outset. But the need to maintain nutrient synergy can make things difficult here. When you can get large amounts of Vitamin A and Vitamin D3 easily from liver and supplements, it becomes difficult to balance this all with natural levels of Vitamin K2 (as well as various minerals).

Loading high amounts of Vitamin D3 initially might work for some people. But these nutrients are not a high school science experiment. Their chief function (calcium metabolism) can be accelerated aggressively enough to cause issues if they become unbalanced.

I don't want to scare people away from obtaining higher amounts to start. This is why I always suggest getting a blood test. This will let you know if you are, in fact, severely deficient. If so, it could mean that loading up will be more beneficial than the potential downside of throwing off your nutrient synergy. If not, you may be better off sticking with normal recommended consumption levels.

The Role of Fat

Before we move on to the other micronutrients you need, I want to first discuss fat in general. Make no mistake: Fat is a macronutrient — not one of the micronutrients we are discussing here. Nevertheless, it is essential to understand its role in metabolism and optimal human health overall. Vitamin A, Vitamin K2, and Vitamin D3 are all fat-soluble vitamins. It's right there in the name. Your diet needs to have adequate fat for these nutrients to do their job.

First Nation Alaskans on carnivorous diets used to obtain around 80% of their calories from fat and 20% from protein. This is a simplistic answer to macronutrient ratios, as the sheer variety of foods in all native diets resulted in high variance depending on geographical location. But as long as the indigenous group obtained 45%-65% of its total calories from animal foods, they had adequate nutrition.

Fat-soluble vitamins are named so for a reason. They are contained in the fatty parts of the animal, as well as the organs, rather than the muscle meat. So by consuming most of our calories from high-fat animal foods (including fatty muscle meats like ribeye steak), we are increasing the overall nutrient density in the diet (granted that these are high-quality foods).

Another important reason to focus on fat consumption is what it does in terms of reducing overall food volume. Let's look at an example. If you were to eat a half pound of fat and one pound of protein rather than three pounds of lean protein, you can get the same number of calories without putting so much digestive stress and bulk In your stomach. That's a good thing! It means less work for your stomach, gut, and digestive enzymes while getting the same amount of nutrients (and even more in most cases).

We will talk about this more in later chapters, but the more efficient your digestive system becomes, the less inflammation you will experience and the better you will feel.

And historically, in ancient times, the most important element of fat was always simply survival. It was — and is — the fuel that our bodies can utilize the easiest, and this is a major reason why people don't see success on purely high-protein diets that are low in both carbs and fat.

Yes, the body can utilize energy from protein — but not nearly as efficiently as it can from fats. (The same applies carbohydrates to a lesser extent. This is because certain starches and sugars can stress certain organs and digestive enzymes much more than fat digestion.)

Protein is of course necessary for muscle cell growth. But in the big picture, it is really a demand-driven need and this is dependent on the person's lean body mass. Because I used to be heavily into bodybuilding, even now I still carry around 20 more pounds of muscle mass than an untrained person. This means my body's requirement for protein, just to maintain my current physique, is significant. So instead of consuming 80% of my calories from an energy source (fat), my intake may be skewed more towards protein, shooting for anywhere between 60%-70% of calories from fat and the rest from protein.

This may not be the ratio you personally need. But this is something you can dial in over time and don't need to think about too much at the start. In general, you should be prepared to drastically increase your fat consumption compared to previous eating habits and cut out carbs almost entirely. The important part is to not be afraid of fat. You need it and will want to consume a ton! Because without it, not only will you lack energy, but the fat-soluble vitamins will not be entering the environment they need to work best.

Monthly Nutrient Requirements

There is one last thing to address before we move on: "How much?" What type of intake do you actually need for Vitamins A, K2, D3, and Omega-3s?

You should now understand why the RDAs and DRIs are not always adequate. You can look to these to get some idea of what the figures tend to look like, but in time, sticking with this diet will generally work itself out.

If the food you are consuming is of high quality and your macronutrient ratios are correct, we won't have to worry about meeting vitamin and mineral needs. They will be achieved because the food you eat inherently has the right amount. The best way to figure out how much nutrition you need is based on the fat ratios our indigenous ancestors used: 80% fat and 20% protein combined with the organ-to-muscle-to-fat ratios you would find on an actual animal.

Think about it like this: If you eat 50 pounds of meat and 15 pounds of fat in a month that would be the equivalent yield of maybe one large sheep or goat. If we look at the organ tissue size of the liver, it would likely be anywhere from three to four pounds. A conservative estimate would be one-and-a-half pounds of liver per 30 pounds of meat yield.

This same comparison can be applied to all other organs of the animal, from the brain to the lungs to the spleen to the testicles to the adrenals and on and on and on. By consuming all parts of the animal in ideal ratios we achieve a complete nutrient profile. This is what we would have done in nature.

What gets complicated is when we don't want to eat nose to tail. While I do take it to the extreme personally, I know that asking you to eat lungs is a bit much. And in a modern society, we don't necessarily need to do so. There is plenty of liver to go around.

We can simply try to think about the overall nutrient profile of all the organs and swap in alternatives. A hunter-gatherer would have gotten DHA from brains, but, yes, you can just consume fatty fish or eggs instead. Perhaps you prefer chicken liver to beef liver. If so, just eat more of these smaller varieties rather than one large one from a cow.

Overall, you want to stick to the guidelines, understand which vitamins and nutrients you need, and stay away from the negative foods. But you also don't need to overcomplicate things.

We know that almost all known indigenous groups have gotten the majority of their calories from animal foods. We also know, however, that the exact amounts varied quite a bit by culture and geographic region. Though we don't know exactly how their health may have differed due to dietary choices, physical presence and statue was one difference commonly seen between groups that consumed around two-thirds of their calories from animal foods and groups that consumed up to 85% from animal food.

We have heard stories, for example, about the Mongols in Central Asia being very tall and strong. The Roman legions that invaded the Germanic regions of Europe often said these people were very tall and physically imposing. The Age of Exploration captains who landed in North America were often taken by how great the native population was at hunting, especially in their endurance and speed to chase down game. Throughout time, though just anecdotes, there have always been fascinating tales about the physical condition of indigenous communities.

We don't need to be incredibly precise about everything all the time. Because, for one, we have better access to all these sources than our ancestors. It should be easy to get adequate fat and all the liver we can stomach. As long as you are continually replenishing your stores each week, you will be fine.

Secondly, remember that these are fat-soluble vitamins. You will be holding some in your body. You will be pretty much good to go as long as, each week, you just eat a few hundred grams of liver, consume some high-quality cheese, eat something out of the ocean, and get some sun. Then, throw in some free-range eggs to be safe — along with an overall diet based on high-quality animal foods, including seafood. There are optimal eating habits to strive for, but starting to get real, natural nutrition into your diet doesn't need to be over-complicated.

You do also need to consider past deficiencies, however. If you have been eating a SAD diet forever, you will likely be significantly lacking in all four of these areas. You should not try to make up for decades of poor nutrition overnight. Don't start supplementing like a madman.

But it does mean that you should pay extra attention and not slip up. I have been eating this way for years. If I don't get any liver in for two weeks, it won't be the end of the world. You need to make up for lost time, though. Work at consistency in all areas so that you can move forward on your journey to better health as quickly as possible.

In time, you will start to understand everything involved — including how your body responds — and start to dial everything in with much more precision. You will make up for deficiencies, start to repair your Omega ratios, and start getting all the vitamins and minerals in the right balance.

It will take some time. But just by starting on this path and understanding the concepts discussed so far, you will be way ahead of most people and well on your way to optimal health.

Chapter Four

The Other Nutrients: Understanding and Getting Everything Else You Need

No diet can be complete from a nutritional perspective if it overlooks essential vitamins, minerals, elements, and electrolytes. Eating healthy requires you to pay attention to everything to at least some degree. It all matters.

The reason we started with Vitamin A, Omega 3s, Vitamin K2, and Vitamin D3 is because they are equal parts important, misunderstood, and lacking in most modern diets.

The rest of the main nutrients you need — which will be discussed here — are not necessarily less important. But they will be inherently obtained by anyone who prioritizes the Fundamental Four and eats high-quality animal foods.

Even people on poor diets are probably getting most of these nutrients. Many may not be getting enough. Most people are getting them in the wrong ratio. And almost everyone is getting them from the wrong sources. But it is less likely for people to be missing out entirely on Vitamin B compared to the millions who consume hardly any retinol and avoid the sun like the plague.

Yes, as a rule, fat-soluble vitamins are more vital to key bodily functions and systems than some of the water-soluble vitamins. But don't look at them as lesser. It's just a matter of what you need to prioritize and focus on obtaining on a day-to-day basis. Vitamin C is important, sure. If you only have 10 minutes to get in some nutrition for the day, though, grab a few bites of aged cheese for Vitamin K2 and the extra fat — not an orange.

With that in mind, the following breaks down the best of the rest, adding some clarity and advice about how to get all the other nutrients you need to move closer to optimal health. We won't go into as much depth here, but understand that this is all critical to consume as well.

B Vitamins

Though they are of the water-soluble variety, it is no less vital to get all your B Vitamins. This large group — made up of eight different nutrients also known by names like Thiamine,

Riboflavin, and Niacin — overall plays a role in nervous system function and cell metabolism, including involvement in enzymatic processes in every cell.

This ranges from converting nutrients into energy, acting as antioxidants, cell signaling, DNA production and repair, amino acid metabolism, red blood cell production, and regulation of gene expression. Specifically, Vitamin B12 — which is only found in animal foods — is regarded as vital for neurological function.

Then there is methylation — arguably the most important individual process in the body. This is the process by which methyl groups are added to the DNA molecule, essentially telling your body what it needs to do. Many cellular processes are dependent on methylation: DNA/RNA creation, all stages of development, immune function, detoxification pathways, and energy metabolism, among others. The list really does go on and on.

But there are a few things to note. First, methylation is greatly influenced by Vitamin B consumption, and the process of methylation also produces Glutathione, which is the most important antioxidant in the body. By comparison, it makes the antioxidants found in plant foods seem inconsiderable. Glutathione is capable of preventing cell damage caused by oxidative stress, including damage from free radicals and heavy metals.

B Vitamin: Sources & Preparation

When it comes to B Vitamins, there is some good news for anyone who is already having a tough time keeping all this straight. Although foods like liver and oysters do contain much higher amounts of certain B vitamins, you will mostly achieve your entire requirement for these nutrients just by consuming the same foods we have already discussed.

As long as you're eating high-quality animal foods, and especially if you're making sure to get in good liver and seafood, you don't have to focus that much on this area. If you eat meat, eggs, and raw dairy, you will get most of your B Vitamins. Folate may become an issue if eggs, dairy, or organs are not being consumed, so do keep an eye on that.

Vitamin E

As the only fat-soluble vitamin not previously mentioned, Vitamin E is of course important. Its role in the body is primarily that of an antioxidant, preventing production of reactive oxygen species (excess oxidation) in the diet. This is necessary to keep inflammation low and reduce the risk of disease essentially across the board.

One important note: All nutrients to some degree require others to be absorbed. But in the case of Vitamin E, proper absorption is *heavily* dependent on Vitamin C, Vitamin B3, Selenium, and Glutathione. But rather than playing as some sort of chemist (or a vegan with a blender), most of these will work themselves out if you're eating the Ancestral Indigenous Diet.

Vitamin E: Sources & Preparation

More good news: Vitamin E is inherent to high-quality animal fat, especially eggs and dairy. As with Vitamin C, this fact isn't as widely known as it should be. The amount contained in animal foods isn't low, but the reason plant foods have more by comparison is because of their Omega 6 Polyunsaturated fatty acids (PUFAs). These fats in plants are by nature unstable, so they require more antioxidants to prevent oxidation. And with Vitamin E being an antioxidant, it makes sense that we would have more.

But plant foods aren't necessary to obtain Vitamin E. Eggs, raw dairy, fatty fish, beef fat, marrow, and brain are all excellent sources. And since this list is pretty similar to the foods you will be eating to maintain high levels of Omega-3s, you should be all set as long as you follow the core principles of this diet. Of note: The quality of the food here is paramount. Low-quality meat from feedlot farms doesn't have much Vitamin E.

The only other thing to keep in mind is that it is technically ideal to only lightly cook your egg yolks and fat in general. This will ensure that the Vitamin E content isn't damaged, although this isn't that big of a concern with this nutrient. (It's a good habit in general though, as lighter cooking will also reduce the oxidation of cholesterol.)

Vitamin C

Of all the vitamins we consume, everybody knows the most about Vitamin C. The orange juice lobby alone has spent bank vaults full of money over the decades to make sure every mother and teacher in America is pumping their kids full of sugar water that will supposedly keep them from getting a cold.

But although it has been overhyped and many people pointlessly consume (then pee out) way more than they need, it is of course very necessary for human health. Specifically, Vitamin C is required for collagen synthesis — which makes it a structural component of all connective tissue, blood vessels, tendons, ligaments, cartilage, gums, skin, teeth, and bones. It also plays a role in neurotransmitters and is involved in the metabolism of cholesterol into bile acids.

Vitamin C also plays a role in carbohydrate metabolism. So even when consuming Vitamin C in something like orange juice, the amount of sugar you ingest at the same time is not natural. Wild fruits of the past, like camu camu and kakadu plums, have substantially higher Vitamin C content without the sugar.

And as all the marketing (rightfully) tells you, Vitamin C plays a role in immune function through the generation of T-Cells (which are immune cells). Other vital, but less-discussed, factors are how it serves as an effective antioxidant that reduces damage from free radicals and works to help synthesize carnitine, which is essential for converting fat to energy in cells.

Vitamin C: Sources & Preparation

All meat contains small amounts of Vitamin C. The fresher it is, the more Vitamin C it will have. Certain organs and glands, certain parts of fish (and especially fish eggs), and some raw dairy products are actually quite high in Vitamin C, especially raw milk.

As long as you are eating fresh meat and other animal products that haven't been frozen for very long, you will be fine. If you do find yourself only having access to cuts that were slaughtered a while ago, Vitamin C intake can become a concern.

Fortunately, the solution is quite simple: a whole-food based Vitamin C supplement, like acerola cherry powder. (Herbs like thyme also have some Vitamin C.) While it isn't necessary if food sourcing and preparation is done right, some people decide to rely on supplementation more regularly, or perhaps just at the beginning, just as a psychological safety blanket.

Cutting out all that citrus fruit may make some people uneasy, but don't worry. Even on a carnivore diet, modern life will never be anything like a year-long voyage on a pirate ship. There is not a real risk of getting scurvy if you eat high-quality foods.

Antioxidants

The nutrition world has become obsessed with "antioxidants" and "free-radicals." You can't find an article on nutrition, or even general health, that doesn't mention them, and this trend is being used to sell all sorts of useless supplements that nobody needs. It's a shame because they do have a big role to play, especially as we discussed in terms of Vitamin C, Vitamin E, and Glutathione.

Overall, the two most important things to understand is that the body can only produce so many antioxidants and deal with so much stress. Specifically, we're talking about oxidative stress. All the mechanisms that cause this, and all the reasons that it is so damaging to our bodies, are too much to detail here. But the big takeaway is knowing that all this stress is negative for your health.

From this perspective, improving health can best be achieved by limiting the causes of oxidative stress rather than merely relying on trying to fix it after the fact. This means focusing on keeping the negative things out of your diet as opposed to ingesting "positive" things to repair the damage.

Did you ever hear the story about the old lady that swallowed the fly? Then she ate a spider to fix the problem. Then she swallowed a bird, a cat, and a dog to deal with the new problems each one created. Well, it seems to me, she would have been best off by just never eating that fly to begin with. The same goes for you and foods that cause oxidative stress and inflammation.

If you just cut out all the seed oils and high-carbohydrate crap in your diet, you will not need nearly as much Vitamin E and Vitamin C, let alone concern yourself with devouring fad "superfood" staples like goji berries and kale or expensive supplements that provide few benefits.

There will still be other modern factors — like environmental pollution and electromagnetic frequencies (EMF) — that will cause stress on your body. Some of this is unavoidable. But simply steering clear of the dietary sources will do wonders to keep your oxidative stress levels low.

Some people even talk about stressors as a means to introduce "hormesis," which is when your body can get some supposed benefit by withstanding negative stimuli. But our modern world has plenty of hormesis. There is no need to intentionally induce it.

Minerals, Elements & Electrolytes

Electrolytes are frequently mentioned when discussing the Keto Diet or Carnivore Diet. But despite all the confusion, there is no need to supplement them granted you are following the nutrient-density principles of the Ancestral Indigenous Diet. Mineral intake will be achieved inherently from all the high-quality food sources you are consuming.

One main consideration to remember is that the three key electrolytes — potassium, magnesium, and calcium — are much more bioavailable in their animal form compared to their plant form. While your RDA recommendations and food labels may make you think you aren't consuming enough, that really isn't the case. One pound of meat, for example, contains approximately 1400 mg of potassium, 80 mg of magnesium, and 40 mg of calcium. And, importantly, they are all highly bioavailable forms.

Someone who is consuming one to two pounds of animal foods per day would get far more of these minerals than anyone on a "high nutrient" plant-based diet. On paper, it may seem like you need to eat a whole bag of spinach every day to get the recommended allotment of magnesium, for example. But this is largely because the magnesium in vegetables is largely bound to substances (such as phytates and oxalates) that inhibit mineral absorption. By contrast, the magnesium you get from high-quality beef is almost fully absorbed and put to work in the body. As far as plant foods go, seaweed can be a great food to try for electrolytes as it contains ample potassium, magnesium, and calcium.

Sodium

The one electrolyte not talked about above is sodium, which most people just call salt. It is essential despite its recent reputation for being unhealthy. This fact has become confused largely because there is so much (poor-quality) sodium contained in the processed foods that everybody eats. But in an ancestral, natural diet, you will actually need to be working to get salt into your system.

There are various salts (Himalayan, Celtic salt, generic sea salt), but the point is to get a quality sea salt with nothing added to it. Salt your food to taste and craving. But be mindful that certain salts can be "saltier" than others. It should also be noted that salt is very subjective. Some people may need large amounts initially (or continuously), while others find they don't need salt hardly at all. This can be observed in indigenous diets as well. Some of them sought after salt. Many of them did not have salt.

Iodine

One aspect of our diet that often goes under the radar is iodine. One way we know that this is important is by understanding that many indigenous people who did not obtain significant iodine from the animal foods they were consuming went out of their way to gather it. This was typically something seen at higher elevations where the grass did not contain enough iodine from the ocean-fueled rainfall.

In modern times, if you consume high-quality dairy and eggs you will generally get enough iodine. Organs like liver also have iodide present, and seafood of course is the best option for iodide. (Seaweed is also great but could come with a pollutant concern.) The high mineral content can also be an issue for people with pre-existing stomach conditions. Iodine levels are directly linked with body temperature. If you eat high-iodine foods and notice your core temperature start to rise, there will be a peak. Once you hit the peak, that hypothetically means you have likely reached your ideal iodine intake.

In the past I have personally used seaweed to increase my iodine levels. But because of the variation in different types of seaweed, I also use Lugol's iodine sometimes. It can be taken either orally or through transdermal delivery on the skin.

Everything Else

I obviously have not discussed every nutrient here. There are many minerals that could be discussed, and depending on past diet and lifestyle, you may run into issues in the long run related to any of them.

Some people may have high ferritin (iron) levels from consuming fortified breads and cereals their whole lives. Many people have a copper-to-zinc ratio imbalance (ideally above 8:1 zinc to copper), being deficient in either copper or zinc. Although a hair mineral analysis is not a fully accurate tool, it may give you a starting point when it comes to understanding your levels.

For instance, if you're deficient in copper and iron, maybe you would make sure to eat more liver initially. On the other hand, if you're overloaded with zinc, which meat is very high in, maybe you opt for fish like salmon or clams that have lower zinc, with higher copper.

The reason you don't want to start worrying about specific minerals, electrolytes, or supplementing, however, is because they are thrown out of balance incredibly easily. If you get a hair mineral analysis and know for certain that you can safely supplement and monitor your levels, that is an option. But nature did not intend for us to take electrolyte powders and metal supplements every day.

In general, most of the other nutrients will work themselves out. I know I keep saying this. But it's the truth. You will have enough to worry about when it comes to the big-ticket items. Focus on those and eat in a natural way to help ensure that you are obtaining Vitamin A, Vitamin D3, and Vitamin K2 as well. I really want to emphasize nutrient synergy. It is very important for optimal health to get these in the right ratios.

But as you fix deficiencies and start dialing in your eating habits, this will all start to even out naturally. Then, a year or two down the line, perhaps you can start concerning yourself more with precise intakes of Selenium, Manganese, Boron, and other trace minerals by isolating specific foods for certain nutrients.

Chapter Five

Chronic Inflammation: How to Avoid the Silent Killer

So far, we have discussed all the nutrients we need. Now it is time to talk about the one big thing you need to avoid: inflammation. After achieving nutrient density, this is the second big goal of the Ancestral Indigenous Diet.

By now, most people have heard the warnings to avoid this so-called "silent killer." But like so many health and nutrition topics, hearing about something doesn't mean understanding it. There is a ton of confusion out there.

For this reason, we need to start with a pretty basic question: First off, what is inflammation? In an overall biological sense, inflammation is natural and a very good thing. It is our body's way of trying to fix a problem by ramping up the production of white blood cells and kickstarting other healing mechanisms. It is an immune system response to make us better.

This good inflammation — "acute inflammation" — happens after we get a cut on our arm, for example. You want this to happen. Without this immune response, people might die from a small scrape.

But when the nature of the "problem" that the immune system is trying to fix isn't clear, our body can overreact. Rather than targeting a specific problem, the body initiates a low-level immune response that isn't actually necessary, can cause discomfort, and may harm our internal systems.

The Standard American Diet (SAD) leaves people in a constant state of inflammation. This is why so many people see immediate benefits from simply not eating and the modern trend of Intermittent Fasting is gaining popularity. If you can feel the best you've felt in years simply by avoiding a few of your typical meals, it really says something about how poisonous modern food is.

Think about the typical foods people eat every day: cereal with low-fat milk for breakfast, a ham sandwich for lunch, and pizza for dinner. Each of these meals causes an inflammatory response in your body to some degree.

Let's look at just breakfast. The cereal likely has high sugar content and is full of "anti-nutrients" that can cause problems ranging from "leaky gut" to the malabsorption of minerals in the intestines. These industrial farmed grains were also sprayed with dangerous agrochemicals in the form of herbicides like glyphosate and any number of pesticides and additives that are included in so many processed foods.

The milk, because it has been pasteurized and homogenized, is likely rancid and definitely lacking any of the desirable nutrients found in raw, grass-fed dairy. Plus, like the cereal, it is high in sugar and also triggers an insulin response that, over time, can lead to the "chronic inflammation" that most people live with constantly throughout their digestive system and, really, their whole body.

The related mechanisms, problems, and causes of "chronic inflammation" are too complex to detail in full here. But what you need to know is that eating certain foods — including most of the foods listed in the common daily meals above — leads to inflammation. And this can be quite bad for our gut and other organs, including our heart.

The result is a dysfunctional internal system that is effectively attacking the substances that we are eating, and this becomes associated with many negative issues you've likely heard about, from "oxidation" and "free radicals" to "leaky gut" and "atherosclerosis." Over time, inflammation may even become one of the contributors to diabetes, heart disease, and possibly even cancer.

Inflammation Warning Signs

Knowing all this is great, but how can someone identify chronic inflammation in their own body? Well, if you eat the Standard American Diet, you are likely experiencing it on some level.

The signs are rampant. Rather than seeing them as significant problems, however, most people just learn to live with them. So many Americans constantly experience gas, bloating, upset stomach, diarrhea, heartburn, acid reflux, GERD, mucus buildup, or persistent cough. They think this is just part of life — but it shouldn't be. This is gastric distress caused largely by the food you eat, and it is accompanied by never-ending low-level inflammation in your gut.

Beyond the discomfort, inflammation can generally make you more lethargic, fill your head with brain fog, cause poor memory, and lead to emotional reactiveness. Overall, it can negatively impact how all your internal systems function and sap you of the energy you need to feel good in your daily life.

You shouldn't be medicating against all these symptoms or even just living with them. This is a chronic condition — even if it doesn't seem debilitating. You need to fix the root cause so it all goes away and you can start living a better life. (Speaking of medication, if you are taking one, it's important to understand its metabolism, what it's doing in your body, and how to address that issue or deal with any potential consequences.)

The biggest issue for many people is that they don't even realize there's a problem. Because if you don't ever experience the difference between this way of life — the default state for most people — and a very-low-inflammation diet, then you won't ever realize how bad your current diet is.

Our society normalized terrible health so much that millions of people take a pill every day just to alleviate gastrointestinal diseases that are by and large solely due to an unnatural diet. Walking around with Tums and Nexium in your pocket isn't normal! You are sick!

If you don't fix the real issue, you will never know just how good you are supposed to feel. You will never know actual human "normal."

Beyond the energy boost and mental clarity, many people find they can sleep less and still function fine after reducing inflammation to near zero. They feel fewer aches and pains in joints and muscles. And they have almost none of the gastric problems that they once thought were just a part of eating.

Sugar and the SAD Reality

There are so many foods and dietary habits that cause low-level inflammation. We cannot discuss them all. But there is one big culprit that most people consume way too much of every single day.

Let's just look at sugar, perhaps the most problematic staple of the SAD diet. It can contribute to many inflammatory and inflammatory-adjacent issues, including insulin resistance, leaky gut, dysbiosis, and general weight gain.

It goes without saying that you want to avoid all these issues, which are commonly seen by people on the SAD eating habits like those we discussed in the example above.

Remember: We've only dealt with breakfast so far. If that was the only "bad" meal you ate all year, you would probably be fine. But most people follow the bad with more bad — meal after meal every day for weeks, months, years, and even decades. This compounds what could be a minor concern over and over and over again until the condition is chronic.

The bread in the sandwich has similar properties to the cereal. That's inflammatory. The ham is likely from pigs that were fed a high Omega-6 diet that throws off the ratio of Omega-6 to Omega-3 fats in the body. That's inflammatory. The deli meat, like so many processed foods that have 50 ingredients on the label, is also likely full of additives and chemicals. That's inflammatory. The mayonnaise or various other condiments probably have added hydrogenated vegetable oils — one of the most detrimental foods to consume — that are highly oxidized Omega-6 fats. That's inflammatory.

The body triggers an immune response whenever these fats end up in the bloodstream. Over time, your body will become composed of linoleic acid (a type of Omega-6 fat). And when cholesterol becomes composed of linoleic acid, it can get inflamed in the arteries. This inflammation, more than just the mere presence of cholesterol itself, may be what is causing so many strokes and heart attacks in the United States.

But the meals we have used as examples are all junk food, you might say. What about "healthier" options? Surely they are fine? Right?

Chicken breast and rice might not seem so bad from an inflammation perspective. Because they are so lean, even grain-fed chickens aren't adding much in the way of Omega-6 fatty acids. But they probably have hormones and antibiotics that aren't great to ingest. And what type of rice are you eating? With all the attention now paid to the glycemic index, most people now know that white rice breaks down quickly, so maybe you will avoid it and the related insulin response. Whole-grain rice, however, comes with lectins that can trigger an immune response, among other issues. And any type probably is laced with pollutants, arsenic, and agrochemicals.

This sure is a lot to keep track of. And don't forget the primary goal of our diet. Beyond everything else, your "healthy" lunch is still missing the most important thing we need: nutrients.

Hoping Vitamins Will Protect You

If nutrient density is the first goal of the diet, the second is removing inflammation. Of course, you could try to figure out what foods your body tolerates and which ones you don't through a process of elimination. But the easiest way is to simply remove everything that doesn't serve a purpose and then reintroduce foods one at a time.

This is one of the primary reasons I have chosen to eat carnivore and stick to animal foods. First off, I know this gives my immune system all the vitamins and nutrients it needs to operate optimally. This means that my body is much more capable of handling any inflammation that does occur. Because even if I eat perfectly, I still live in New York and am exposed to contaminants and pollution that my body has to deal with. How can it handle all that if it's so busy fighting off all the perceived attacks it is so worried about from sugars, lectins, and other issues related to leaky gut?

There is one anecdote that helps explain my mentality on all this. I once went through a phase where I ate liver everyday with butter. Generally, butter causes me to break out. In some capacity, there is a combination of nutrients and bacteria in every individual's microbiome that allows different people to tolerate different foods. Combined with allergies and other issues, this means that you and I may react very differently to certain things we eat. The fat particles in butter can be hard to digest for some, and were likely giving me leaky gut.

I'm not fully sure about the science of it all. But my theory was that, even though I am allergic to butter, consuming it alongside such a high-vitamin food would prevent me from getting acne. It worked! The Vitamin A from liver, in particular, seems to always help eliminate acne whenever I have a breakout.

This is still kind of bit stupid though. The better idea — which I quickly learned — was to simply eliminate the butter and eat liver by itself. I can get all the nutrients available from butter in another way. So why am I torturing myself and looking for anecdotes to an allergy that I can just avoid in the first place

The Elimination Protocol: Cut It Out

Over the past decade, the "health and wellness" community has been focused more and more on antioxidants. Study after study tries to determine which foods and plants we can eat to lower the levels of oxidative stress that cause inflammation, accelerate aging, and generally harm our health. People are now stuffing their faces with blueberries, turmeric, and goji berries — even chocolate and wine — in hopes of repairing themselves.

That's all fine and good. But it seems to me that there's an even better solution. Rather than looking for magic superfoods that will help reverse the damage — like I once did with liver to cure my acne — why not just stop consuming the things that we know cause oxidative stress and inflammation in the first place?

At some level, everything you ever eat puts some stress on the body. (This is a main reason why fasting can be so beneficial.) But certain foods — like grass-fed, hormone- and antibiotic-free beef — cause almost no inflammation. Omega-3 fatty acids also don't cause nearly the same immune-system response as the Omega-6 fatty acids that people shovel into their mouths all day long.

It's almost too obvious. The best way to protect yourself from the dangers of inflammation would be to never eat. But that is unrealistic for any human who wants to remain alive.

The second-best way, then, is to stop eating inflammatory foods. If you can get all the nutrients you need from animal foods and avoid all the inflammation you don't want, doesn't it just make sense to stick to these foods? Or is that kale and spinach smoothie just too delicious to give up?

If you don't actually need it for nutrition — and it's not even good for you — the solution is simple: Cut it out. What you don't eat can't hurt you.

Chapter Six

Plant Food Myths: Why Fruits, Vegetables, and Grains Aren't Necessary

Oatmeal is a common part of the modern diet and one deemed as a bona fide health food by nutritionists across the world. This is despite the fact that it is usually sold in single-serving packets mixed with apple cinnamon or brown maple sugar flavor concoctions. Once reserved for vegetarian stores, oat milk has also exploded on the scene and forms the base for millions of vegan Oatly oatmilk smoothies every day.

In these forms, it's hard to find anything good to say about this grain. But it has long had a place in the human diet — if prepared properly. The way you make your oatmeal can make all the difference between your breakfast being a nourishing energy source or a potentially inflammatory food to avoid.

Let's explore this with a little history lesson. Oatmeal has been a staple in Scotland since before the place was even called Scotland. After arriving in the British Isles, likely during the Iron Age, and becoming part of the traditional Gaelic culture in the region, the grain has become synonymous with these people.

When Samuel Johnson wrote the Dictionary of the English Language in 1755, he included this in his definition of oats: "A grain, which in England is generally given to horses, but in Scotland supports the people." (Some local humor can be seen in a popular response: "That's why England has such fine horses and Scotland such fine men.")

Oats became the preferred grain here because they grew well in the wet, cold, harsh climate of these northern highlands. They also happened to be a good choice due to their relatively higher caloric and fat content compared to other options at the time like bulgur wheat, buckwheat, rye, sorghum, and barley, according to the Whole Grains Council. In times of scarcity, oats could be stretched just that much further.

Today you can even buy "Scottish Oats" all across the world, although even this steel-cut variety differs greatly from the raw "groats" that were used historically. Generally, you won't find these in your local supermarket, and even the hippies that may opt for this type fail to cook them properly in line with the traditional preparation method.

In a process that dentist Weston Price observed during his trip to the isolated Isles of Lewis and Harris almost a century ago, the not-yet-modernized Gaelic communities — who we wrote had "teeth of unusual perfection" and "a physique that rivals that found in almost any place in the world" — relied heavily on fermentation to create their porridge.

Among those still living a traditional lifestyle and eating the traditional way, oats were a main energy source to complement a diet otherwise full of fish, lobster, crabs, oysters, and clams. "An important and highly relished article of diet has been baked cod's head stuffed with chopped cod's liver and oatmeal," wrote Price in his classic book *Nutrition and Physical Degeneration*. He reported that "fruits are practically unknown" and that even dairy was limited.

Another book, *The Scots Kitchen*, written by Florence Marian McNeill in 1929, helps explain the traditional process of turning raw oats into something known to these people as "sughan" (or "sowans" in English). First, the full groat would be milled and ground into husks called "sids." These would then be soaked in water for seven days. Sometimes they would soak the mixture even longer. After that long bath, the sids would then be tossed aside and the cloudy water was reserved to rest for a few more days. The floating remnants — forming something of a cloudy sediment — would settle over time in the container. This substance is what would become the sowans.

Through generations of passed-on wisdom, these Gaelic communities had learned that this process was a great way to extract all the nutrition from the grain while discarding the negative parts that were hard to digest and generally detrimental to consume. The substance left over "contains practically all the nutritious properties of the oatmeal in its most easily digested form," wrote McNeill. In modern terminology, we would say this method was a way to make the nutrients more "bioavailable" to our bodies.

To actually prepare the meal into its final sowans form, they would then heat it up, adding salt and dairy (raw cream or milk most of the time). The result was a meal both high in calories from the grains and rich in vitamins and other nutrients from the added raw milk fat.

The Role of Oats in the Gaelic Diet

This classic dish can be traced back to an ancient culture and perfectly illustrates the historic role that plant foods have played in the human diet. Even after the advent of livestock, it was difficult to procure a community's worth of all the calories from animals. There were only so many cows, and any of them could get sick and die at a moment's notice from a mysterious illness sent by the gods.

Besides, these domesticated animals didn't really resemble modern cattle. At least not functionally. The cows these old Gaelic people would have raised would have produced a fraction of the milk that today's super cows pump out. The increase in just the last century alone has been staggering. Genetic selection, breeding, farm science, and chemicals have forever changed husbandry into a profit-motivated industry.

In 1900, according to a study from the Journal of Dairy Sciences, a dairy cow in the United States could be expected to produce an average of around 11 pounds of milk per day. By 1950, this number was up to 14.6 pounds, and it nearly doubled to 28.4 pounds each day by 1975, per USDA figures. But they were just getting started. In 2000, the average cow would produce 49.9 pounds per day — and the top-performers would do way better than that.

"Production as high as 60 kilograms (132 pounds) per day is not uncommon," stated the Journal of Dairy Sciences paper about modern high-producing cows. "In fact, the current world-record Holstein produced more than 30,000 kilograms (72,752 pounds) of milk in a year. That's almost 90 kilograms (198 pounds) per day on average — enough to feed more than 100 people."

The people who once lived in modern-day Scotland — even in the best seasons — never had access to the animal products we take for granted today. Living with scarcity, it only made sense to stretch everything as far as possible.

That was likely the inspiration for this porridge dish that nobody in today's society would ever expend so much effort to make. As labor intensive as this process was, the caloric expenditure in doing so was probably comparable to gathering wild plant foods and it was a much more certain way to feed yourself.

But they knew that whole grains were not worth eating in their natural form. So they went through all this to make the sowans. In a pure nutritional sense, they would have been fine just drinking raw cream and eating cheese. But it wouldn't last as long for the community or the individual family.

Thus, a great compromise: Use half the dairy and mix it into some long-prepared oats. You preserve your resources, get adequate nutrition, and fuel up with carbs for enough energy to make it until tomorrow. There's even an added bonus to this survival strategy: It tastes great!

Understanding and Avoiding Anti-Nutrients

There was one other great reason to put so much effort into oatmeal preparation. Without even knowing the science behind it, they had also gone to great lengths to remove most the dreaded "anti-nutrients" contained in the grains.

This was something they surely learned over time. It is likely that they observed negative effects if they consume oats prepared in other ways. Maybe the issues were just digestive. Maybe it was just feeling bad or lacking energy. Or perhaps they saw dental problems, suffered skeletal issues, or even stunted development.

Either way, we can forgive the Gaelic people living centuries ago for not knowing the term "anti-nutrients." But it's really, really strange that almost nobody today talks about it either.

What exactly are antinutrients? In the most basic terms, anti-nutrients are any negative substances found in plant foods that can inhibit certain processes in the body, such as digestive enzymes or mineral absorption, and in turn impair metabolic function.

In something closer to normal English, they are compounds that make the "paper value" of minerals and vitamins in many grains and vegetables misleading. The numbers and RDA percentages you see on the bag of veggies may look promising. But antinutrients, among other factors, mean your body probably isn't going to ever use a lot of it. So does it really matter how much magnesium is technically in a pound of spinach if your gut is incapable of ever absorbing it?

Gluten, a protein in many grains that some people can't tolerate, is the one anti-nutrient that has become well known. Some cereals also contain other proteins, such as avenins (in oats) and gliadin (in wheat), that can cause digestive issues. Then there are the lectins (found in high levels in legumes), oxalates (common in green vegetables), and many others that are widespread in modern diets.

As a rule, you don't want to be consuming these. They are believed to have evolved as something of a defense mechanism for plants. Think of it like this: Cheetahs got really fast to avoid being eaten. Turtles weren't so lucky in that department, but they have survived with strong armor. Cobras have poisonous venom and long fangs.

Plants, on the other hand, can't move or physically protect themselves very well. So they turned to chemistry and started producing substances that can harm anything that eats them. Insects and other smaller animals can face significant problems if they consume too many.

There have even been documented cases of people dying from toxicity caused by glycoalkaloids in sprouted potatoes. But for humans, anti-nutrients historically have been more of a complication. They can cause an inflammatory response in our digestive systems, disrupt the microbiome in our intestines, and lead to other chronic problems.

In high enough amounts, they may even contribute to problems like "leaky gut" syndrome (permeability of the epithelial lining), that damages the walls of our small intestine badly enough to allow larger particles to pass through into our bloodstream. These substances are not meant to exit the gut this way. So it is speculated that this can cause a whole host of issues and promote chronic inflammation because it triggers our immune system to start fighting what it sees as a foreign invasive.

These and other concerns are a large reason why the Ancestral Indigenous Diet includes no plant foods. In the future — after you fix years of health problems caused by a bad diet — if high-quality organic plant foods are accessible, incorporating them and gauging your individual tolerance could be a hypothetical goal. But, simply put, you don't actually need them for nutrition. They are often inflammatory. And they may cause other types of damage in our gut.

It is not within the scope of this book to break down all the complex science associated with these compounds or participate in the endless debate about how serious all the potential effects might be. There are countless studies across dozens of peer-reviewed journals that have been analyzing all this for years.

But there are undoubtedly some real concerns to consider. So the following breakdown offers a list of a few of the most common anti-nutrients, where they are typically found, and why they might be problematic.

Phytic Acid / Oxalates

Found in: grains, legumes, greens, nuts, seeds

While phytic acid (phytates) and oxalates are different in nature, they are spoken about together quite frequently in a vegetarian/vegan diet because they both inhibit the absorption of various minerals. They are unique from one another scientifically but the main difference for our purposes is that phytic acid is found in grains, legumes, nuts, and seeds, while oxalates are in both greens and legumes.

Phytic acid inhibits the absorption of phosphorus, calcium, copper, iron, magnesium, zinc, and manganese. The degree of disruption can be as high as 80% (for phosphorus and calcium) or 40% (manganese) depending upon the mineral. Oxalates are primarily associated with inhibiting the uptake of calcium, iron, and magnesium (by binding to these minerals). Because these two ant-nutrients often overlap so greatly in vegan/vegetarian diets where intake is so high (and animal sources don't exist), this is one reason that anemia (iron deficiency) is so common.

Glucosinolates

Found in: cruciferous vegetables, including broccoli, cauliflower, kale, cabbage, brussels sprouts

Glucosinolates are known to be goitrogens (meaning that they can potentially encourage the growth of goiters when consumed in large amounts) and have been shown in some animal studies to lead to free radicals. They also go hand in hand with the presence of isothiocyanate, which can stimulate detoxification enzymes (creating an inflammatory response), interfere with DNA segregation (leading to cell death), and inhibit both iodine uptake and thyroid hormone. Beyond this, glucosinolates consumption is associated with indoles (inhibiting ATP energy metabolism) and nitriles (stimulating detoxification enzymes).

These substances are found in high volumes in cruciferous vegetables, which include broccoli, cauliflower, cabbage, kale, and brussels sprouts. Interestingly, none of these are naturally occurring but can all be traced back to a singular ancestor — wild mustard — and only exist as different varieties now due to artificial selection made by farmers over the past few thousand years. One means of reducing glucosinolates is to boil vegetables, but few people do that before consuming any of the popular cruciferous veggies.

Gluten

Found in: wheat, rye, barley, malt, yeast (and all the processed variants of these grains)

As the most well-known anti-nutrient, gluten has gotten a bad wrap even beyond its role in celiac disease — and this is one piece on modern health advice that they actually got correct. It's good to avoid no matter how much of an obvious intolerance you have, especially because it is an enzyme inhibitor. Without getting too long-winded, anything that inhibits enzymes will impair digestive function. If your body isn't producing the proper enzymes (or enough of them), your food can essentially just sit there in your stomach and ferment rather than being broken down.

This can cause damage to cells, contribute to leaky gut, become associated with autoimmune diseases, or promote the growth of bad gut bacteria. Among the more outward symptoms, some have severe allergies (celiac disease) while others report cognitive problems (including poor memory), joint pain, headaches, and fatigue. Even in the best scenario, it is among the compounds in plants that can just cause excessive gas and farts, as we see in so many vegans who flood their guts with anti-nutrients 24/7.

Isoflavones

Found in: soy, peanuts, chickpeas, fava beans, kudzu, alfalfa

The main concern of isoflavones is its role a phytoestrogen, which may be associated with reduced fertility (shown in studies on rats), cell death (in embryos), early puberty in women, and irregular menstrual cycle. On a personal note, I blame the heavy concentration of isoflavones in the soy formula I was fed as an infant for a lot of the allergies and food tolerance problems that I have faced. Even more than the others, this may be seen as a poison that negatively alters our hormones and system function overall.

Lectins

Found in: legumes, grains, vegetables, oils, dairy

Because lectins are attracted to the sugar in cells, they can damage the intestines and cause joint pain. While some people can tolerate these better than others, along with gluten and saponins, lectins bind to many cells in the bonds and are believed to be among the main anti-nutrients that contribute to leaky gut syndrome. And interactions with lectins contained in dairy, and the homogenization process, explain why many people have issues with store bought conventional dairy. In many cases, however, they can be reduced significantly through fermentation or soaking.

Glycoalkaloids – Solanine and Chaconine

Found in: nightshades (tomato, bell pepper, chili pepper, potato, eggplant)

Solanine and chaconine are two compounds that are known as glycoalkaloids and have some negative effects. Both can inhibit the nerve-synapse enzyme acetylcholinesterase, and solanines are the primary anti-nutrient found in nightshades. Also known to disrupt cell membranes (by increasing the concentration of potassium in the cytoplasm), solanines can be found in any part of the plant (leaves, fruit, and tubers) and are so abundant in the flowering, above-ground part of the potato that are deemed unfit for human consumption. The amount of solanines found in potatoes, for example, can vary greatly depending upon the specific variety, how they were grown, and the manner in which they were stored.

Saponins

Found in: soy, chickpeas, asparagus, onions, garlic, quinoa, oats, tea

Though sometimes found in different foods, saponins have similar effects to lectins and are another potential problem for the gut, specifically the intestinal lining. They can also damage red blood cells inhibit both enzymes and thyroid function, and introduce something of a "foaming property" that can damage cells. As with lectins, these can be reduced through fermentation and soaking.

Other Anti-Nutrients

This isn't a science textbook and I imagine many of you have already skipped over all these descriptions. That is understandable but the main message is to understand that there are certain anti-nutrients that should be avoided in large amounts and that (as we'll see more below) there are various preparation methods that should be used to reduce the anti-nutrient content in many foods.

A few of the others to keep a look out for negative or related compounds such as lignans, alpha amylase inhibitors, protease inhibitors, sulphites, tannins, biogenic/vasoactive amines, mycotoxins, aflatoxins, salicylates. Some of these occur due to handling and storage of plant foods (rather than being inherent to them), and the evidence for real harm may not be overwhelming at this point. But these are other compounds that we may want to keep an eye on.

Traditional Preparation Methods

The fascinating history of Gaelic oats is just one anecdote. All across the world, indigenous communities have used extensive preparation methods for the grains and other plant foods they consumed. Fermentation lasting days or even weeks was often a major part of this.

Along with other work to turn harsh cereal seeds into edible food (including milling, prolonged soaking, or germination), it was all very laborious and time consuming. But for ancient people who were building societies and struggling to find enough calories to survive, it was well worth the effort.

Especially in one case: beer. While ancient cultures didn't have anything like our modern IPAs, almost every grain-consuming culture has some sort of fermented beverage tradition. Some were more alcoholic than others. Both the Inca society that came to dominate the Andes in South America and many different indigenous groups in the Amazon made versions of "chicha," which was typically made from corn in the mountains and cassava (yuca) in the jungle. And unlike the adult beverages of today, these drinks were made with very high quality grains and used natural wild yeast cultures to ferment, giving them a unique probiotic profile.

Sourdough bread is probably the most famous traditional grain preparation. It relies on a long fermentation process of the starter culture that, through the presence of lactic acid bacteria (lactobacillus), significantly reduces phytate levels in the final bread. Until the development of modern yeasts, this was the traditional method of bread-making for thousands of years in places like the Lötschental Valley in Switzerland, where people lived in great health while mainly consuming cheese and rye bread.

A 2001 study in the Journal of Agricultural and Food Chemistry found that sourdough fermentation can reduce phytate content by 62%. And if the bran was then incubated with microorganisms before baking the bread, the reduction could be as high as 90%. The result is a significantly increased "solubility" of phosphorus and magnesium. Translation: They become easier for the body to absorb, meaning more bioavailable.

Sprouting is another traditional method used to reduce antinutrient content. Modern studies have shown an 88.3% reduction in phytate content "when germinated pearl millet sprouts were fermented" with various bacteria cultures for 72 hours and confirmed that soaking both cereals and beans can be "quite effective for reduction of phytic acid as well as consequent increase in mineral bioavailability."

Unlike modern scientists working in a lab, people living 1,000 years ago in northern Scotland, the Andean Altiplano, or the Swiss Alps didn't know the complicated chemistry and biology behind why fermenting and soaking worked. But they understood the importance of it. They knew that they were healthier and they knew they felt better if they used these methods to produce their food. It was probably so ingrained in their culture that they didn't even think about it. To them, this was just the way these items had to be prepared for humans to eat them.

This is definitely not the case today. People spend almost no time preparing their grains properly. They assume everything is ready to eat out of the bag and then load up — day after day after day — at every meal.

And this is despite the fact that today's grains have been bioengineered to maximize factors like yield and drought resistance at the expense of nutrition. They generally have far less protein. By comparison, some traditional ancient grains, such as einkorn wheat, were higher in protein and fat as well as nutrients like Vitamin B2, potassium, phosphorous, and carotenoids, according to a study published by Purdue University's Center for New Crops & Plant Products. We should also note that this doesn't even take into account the vastly higher mineral content of the soil before the rise of industrial agriculture that has made today's plant foods even less nutritious.

When you add it all up, and you take away the traditional — and necessary — preparation methods, it's clear that all the people today are getting far fewer positives and many more negatives when they eat plant foods.

Ambers Waves of Mold

Maize — the forefather to our modern corn and base of their iconic tortillas — was eaten extensively by the Maya and many ancient cultures in modern-day Mexico and Central America. And like their Gaelic brothers across the Atlantic, they too went to great lengths to get the most out of their favored grain.

"The Maize was prepared by boiling or soaking it in lime water and then draining it in a gourd colander," wrote Elizabeth P. Benson's in her book The Maya World. "While it was still wet, it was ground on a metate — as small stone table — with a *mano*, a cylindrical handstone. The resulting paste was most commonly mixed with water to make *pozole*, a thin gruel, or formed into cakes, the still-familiar tortillas, which were roasted on a flat pottery griddle and eaten with beans or chili."

This alkaline soaking process, now known as nixtamalization, was useful for two reasons. Most importantly, it removed the presence of potentially deadly aflatoxins caused by certain strains of mold. And it may also have helped free up the Vitamin B3 (niacin) that is naturally in a "bound form" in maize. "It is possible that lime treatment followed by cooking makes the niacin more available or perhaps it improves the amino acid balance," wrote Michael C. Latham in the book Human Nutrition in the Developing World.

Getting Vitamin B3 was not a nice benefit to add a little extra nutrition to a food mainly consumed for energy. But this wasn't nearly as critical as avoiding aflatoxins — which can literally kill you. Death only happens in severe cases of acute poisoning, of course. But the World Health Organization warns that "long-term exposure can have serious health consequences" because aflatoxins are "potent carcinogens and may affect all organ systems" or "cause immunosuppression."

Because of this, and more so the risk of a truly deadly outbreak, the FDA mandates strict testing and limits the maximum acceptable level in crops today at 20 parts per billion (ppb) in food intended for use by humans. That upper allowable limit jumps to 300 ppb for feed that will be used to finish beef cattle.

You may notice, however, that neither of these numbers are zero — despite the fact that "frequent aflatoxin B1 exposure accelerates inflammatory responses via regulation of cytokine gene expression," according to a 2017 study in Frontiers in Microbiology.

Maybe those Maya were on to something after all, ya think? When we step away from indigenous food preparations, bad things seem to happen.

Pesticides, Unnatural Crops, and Modern Access

While everything discussed here so far is definitely a real concern, the anti-nutrient threat admittedly can be overblown at times. This is especially true when it comes to the online carnivore community. Without really researching or comprehending the underlying science, many leading advocates of the Carnivore Diet will simply say, "gotta stay away from those damn oxalates, man," as an excuse to sit around eating cheap, grain-fed ribeye steak all day.

Without doubt, flooding your gut with anti-nutrients at every single meal can be detrimental. This is particularly true if you're a vegan or otherwise struggle to get vital nutrients in the first place. The problem of impaired vitamin and mineral absorption is negative for anyone — but it becomes that much worse when you are constantly low or deficient in the true building blocks of health.

That said, anti-nutrients are not going to kill you. Really, compared to all the herbicides, pesticides, and other pollutants coating so many vegetables and plant foods today, this may all be small potatoes.

So what's the real best reason to avoid plant foods? To me, you shouldn't be consuming this stuff because of what we're spraying on it. Before everything else, you need to ask yourself whether your enjoyment of plant foods is worth ingesting poison.

Perhaps if you know a local farmer or you trust in the nation's (poorly regulated) organic labeling standards, you may be able to avoid the worst of the industrial agrochemical contamination. But you're still dealing with the inflammatory properties of modern grains. Then there is the ongoing degradation of soil quality that leaves more and more of these foods devoid of much mineral content to begin with. And, yes, once again, you don't want to be consuming all these anti-nutrients.

Even in the best scenarios, we're still usually talking about a highly bioengineered plant food that was modified greatly over the centuries to no longer resemble anything our ancestors could have found in nature. I'm not even talking about the modern GMO fear.

You should never confuse the modern crops, like broccoli and tomatoes, in our supermarkets with the wild plant foods that humans ate tens of thousands of years ago. These items largely didn't exist in anything resembling their current form. Plus, anyone living far away from the equator never would have been eating fruits and vegetables all that often in the first place. The ground was frozen solid for half the year!

Today, you may be able to fly in avocados from Mexico and ship açaí berries from Brazil to keep your pantry stocked all year long. But there is no way people living in northern Europe were consuming vegetables for months on end in ancient times. So, if we didn't evolve with these foods, why should we eat them now?

Fruit is even worse. Modern versions have been bred and cultivated over time to be bigger and sweeter with fewer seeds than anything that ever would have existed naturally. And while some people whose ancestors evolved in more tropical climates, where fruit was more abundant, may tolerate fruit sugars better than those who hail from Nordic vikings, you have to remember that consuming the foods in large amounts still may have been unlikely during our evolution.

Over time, tools may have helped us get more of these sweet treats. But, by and large, the other animals living in the Amazon, for example, would be getting to this fruit before humans could. Everything from monkeys and other tree-dwelling mammals to high-flying birds and bats were always much more adept than us as procuring fruit way up in a tree.

The energy it took to outfox a gibbon for a primitive orange would hardly be worth the caloric benefit — especially when you remember that an ancient orange was 80% seeds and much lower in fructose than the hybrid-engineered crops today. Why waste all that time and energy for a little sugar when you could just hunt the monkey itself and feast for days?

Anti-Nutrients: Compounding the Real Problem

There is one more key thing to consider when it comes to plant foods: Every indigenous group that consumed plant foods in significant quantities did so not for nutrition but for energy. The move toward agriculture and crops was to obtain calories, as we saw when Gaelic ancestors made their dairy last longer by mixing it with oats.

Think about a fishing community tens of thousands of years ago that subsisted largely by eating a lean catch like bass. Maybe they managed to pull in enough for every member of the group to eat a kilogram (2.2 pounds) of fish per day. If they ate all the organs as well, they would be doing great as far as achieving most of their nutritional needs.

But that's still less than 2,000 calories per day for people who are much more active than we are today. They would need more energy. And it would have been a great benefit to forage for starchy tubers or cultivate wild rice to make up the difference. Even if they could get enough animal protein, it was probably always challenging to find enough animal fat.

Today, conventional wisdom has flooded our brains with the idea that greens and tomatoes are full of nutrients. But they lack all of the fat-soluble vitamins and many other key components we need. And as we now know, in their attempt to use these resources for their caloric needs, traditional cultures also had special preparation methods that removed, or at least limited the negative effects of, these anti-nutrients and other inflammatory aspects.

I want to be fully honest with you here. A few bowls of rice per month, a salad every week, or even an organic apple every day is very unlikely to actually harm your health. This might be true even when it was all grown with gallons of herbicide and pesticide. But if you are getting a high percentage of your calories from plant foods — and most Americans get 60%-70% of their calories from non-animal sources — you need to at the very least reduce the anti-nutrient content.

When you consume grains in large amounts, phytates and phytic acid will inhibit the absorption of minerals in your body. So if you don't ferment the wheat you use to make bread, granted you consume it frequently, you are going to be in very poor health.

But, again, this — and even the pesticides — still really isn't the biggest concern. This isn't the reason that I shake my head every time I see a mom or dad force veganism upon their young, developing child. It still all comes back to the fundamental problem: the lack of animal foods.

If the kid, like many of our grandparents, started off each day with a breakfast of high-quality eggs laid by free-range hens and drank raw milk from a cow grazing on summer pasture, there would be very little problem with them then having an apple a day and eating greens, mashed potatoes, and bread during dinner.

When you take all of this out of the equation, however, the child is getting no significant nutrition — for years on end — and then also compounding that problem with a constant assault of anti-nutrients. This sad reality is what stands out. This is what is destroying our society's health more than the presence of some unfriendly oxalates and lectins.

A quick aside: Consuming too many plant foods, even leafy greens, can disrupt natural ratios of minerals. For example, the ratio of copper and zinc — two antagonistic metals in our body that fight for real estate, so to speak — is much closer to ideal in meat. Daily intake of spinach, which is much higher in copper, can throw this out of whack. Most people actually have a zinc deficiency from prior plant food consumption. The same can happen with potassium and sodium ratios or magnesium and calcium ratios, both of which rely on balance as much as volume to keep our bodies functioning optimally.

Again, we are resilient beings and these ratios being off won't kill us. And, in fairness, eating way too many oysters or way too much liver can throw off ratios too. The thing to remember is that more is not always better. It's much easier to keep everything in harmony with the closer-to-ideal ratios in animal foods rather than by adding in a random assortment of modern, engineered crops that often have strange combinations of minerals and elements.

Because real-world comparisons are sometimes easier to understand than science, Frankie Boy will leave you with one metaphor that may help you put this all together: Think of your body like a car.

Plant foods can do a great job of functioning like gas. While I personally live on a ketogenic metabolism and prefer to use fat as my fuel — which we can call diesel — carbs can work just fine as gasoline to get the automobile from point A to point B. But if gasoline is the only thing you ever put into the car, it will stop functioning properly over time. You're not changing the oil, you're not replacing the brake pads, and you're not putting in new air filters. You are not keeping up on essential maintenance in the form of essential nutrients.

In this state of disrepair, the vehicle may only last a month. Or it may keep on trucking for another three years. But eventually, you can be sure that this car is going to break down.

It may have been working great by just adding gasoline, and gasoline only, for a long time because it's a well-built, highly resilient machine. It will depend upon what type of car it is (much like your genetics) and how long you've been driving it this way (how long ago you stopped consuming high-quality animal nutrition). But, if you keep trying to run it this way without considering the essentials, that car simply cannot last forever.

The Reality About Eating Plants

I don't want to be all doom and gloom about plants. There are plant foods that can have benefits to your health. Studies continue to look at antioxidants and other compounds that may potentially be helpful.

The primary reason that I don't consume any plant foods at all is due to my past Accutane usage and the damage done to my gut. I now have trouble tolerating many foods high in carbohydrates that I consumed frequently in the past. But, admittedly, for a healthy person with a diverse gut microbiome, there may in fact be some aspects that could be positive, especially in terms of feeding certain gut bacteria (although things like milk and honey can also do this).

Ultimately, however, even the best plant foods are really not providing much of anything that someone can't get from animal foods. And there is just so much knowledge required to eat most plant foods the right way. The proper preparation to make even sourdough bread from heirloom grains, not to mention undertaking wild rice fermentation or sowans, is a tall task. And it's often very expensive! So much so that I can afford the highest-quality animal foods but would struggle to ever validate splurging for most rare grains.

Sure, you probably won't see any negative effects from eating a few ounces of macadamia nuts, a handful of wild blueberries, the occasional avocado, or some raw coconut. If you do enjoy these foods and want to consume them once in awhile to add some variety it isn't the end of the world. Maybe it helps you stick to the diet better and stave off feelings of meat-only boredom.

In fact, for someone who struggles to find fatty cuts of grass-fed beef, either financially or because of where they live, eating something like a mashed sweet potato with a half a stick of raw butter could be beneficial on balance. If you're stuck inside all winter with roommates who are sick of you smoking up the apartment by pan-searing steaks, being nice to them and having an avocado and a half-dozen scrambled eggs for dinner won't put you in the hospital.

To be absolutely clear, I am in no way recommending any of this. No plant foods are included as part of the Ancestral Indigenous Diet. But these are just examples to stress the importance of ensuring you consume nutrient-dense animal foods. That, first and foremost, is the goal of this diet much more than preaching philosophically purity or devoutly adhering to some carnivore religion.

One other reason we can't say strict carnivore-eating is the only way to achieve optimal health is the existence of "blue zones." People living in blue zones, a term coined for a few select places where residents tend to live to extraordinarily old ages, definitely consume a wide variety of foods, including many vegetables, fruits, grains, and beans. In this way, they resemble the indigenous groups all throughout history.

Critically, however, the diets of the people living in these special regions — whether in Italy, Japan, Costa Rica, or Greece — have almost always included certain meats, cheeses, seafood, or other locally sourced, high-quality animal foods. Italians in Sardinia eat an average of around 15 pounds of sheep's cheese per year, according to NPR. In Okinawa, Japan, where the most centenarians have been born, they eat fish three times a week plus squid and octopus. And people in Ikaria, Greece, consume a lot of goat's milk and feta cheese.

Consider this: People living in blue zones usually consume around 70% of their calories from plant foods and 30% from animal foods. This is the exact same ratio as the Standard American Diet. What is the difference — in the makeup of the diet and their health? Food quality.

It's also important to note that anybody who has ever lived to be 100 years old grew up in a time before the widespread consumption of modern processed foods. This means that both the animal products and the plant foods they ate in their formative years were coming from much-higher-quality sources than can readily be found today. And toxic herbicides, like glyphosate, had not even been invented. So, unlike most of your options in this century, each piece of lettuce they consumed wasn't laced with industrial poison.

Eating for Modern Times

If you could take a time machine to a Greek island in 1935, eating for health would be a lot easier. You probably couldn't mess it up if you tried. That, unfortunately, is no longer the world we live in. Especially in the United States, you need to understand that access and availability to high-quality foods has grown incredibly scarce.

It's a sad commentary on our society honestly. We have more and more affluence and abundance than ever. But it is harder now for even someone living very comfortably on $100,000 per year to find a good piece of chicken than it was for a poor farmer in the days before World War II.

Just remember: Today, the main purpose of eating any plant food is culinary or psychological enjoyment. You don't need the relatively low amount of nutrients they offer. And in this modern world of abundance, you don't have the excuse of needing extra calories like our ancestors.

But before you even start to talk about including veggies, grains, and nuts, you need to begin learning a lot about avoiding the downsides of inflammation, removing anti-nutrients, understanding which "nuts" and "good fats" to always avoid (like cashews), and where to find heirloom varieties.

The problem with plants is that both the nutrient and anti-nutrient profile of every single food varies so much. What's the anti-nutrient content of white potatoes vs sweet potatoes? White potatoes are nightshades so they are high in solanines. Whereas sweet potatoes are high in oxalates. Learning it all is essentially homework! Good luck trying to live a normal life and keep it all straight.

Gauging the body's response to individual plant foods, and trying to see which antinutrients cause you issues, is a good first step. But, for most people, this is just too time consuming and confusing. And especially if you're coming from a Standard American Diet, you already have enough work to do in terms of understanding why the nutrients from animal foods are so vital and how to source quality products.

That's why my advice is to focus on that. If anything, use your limited time to learn more about the importance of Vitamin A and find a local farm that has high-quality eggs.

If you actually want to get healthy, try to just keep everything as simple as possible while you change your life for the better. You have years of damage to fix. You need to overcome vitamin and nutrient deficiencies and get your Omega ratios back in check. This will take months, if not years, of focused effort toward eating the right animal foods and cutting out the junk.

Don't spend hours each week making sourdough bread with natural cultures and fermenting stone-cut Scottish oats. In general, these can be seen as more-approachable foods to use if introducing your family or friends to better eating habits. Make them einkorn flour cookies, fermented sourdough, or a raw cream cheesecake if you want to spend some effort.

But, personally, you will probably be a lot better off just sticking to the animal foods that we know are the foundation of nutrition. Use the precious time you save to get a little exercise or sit outside in the sunshine.

Eventually, you may want to reintroduce some of these plant foods. With the right information, enough care, and better understanding of how your digestive system reacts to different substances, that should be no problem. Beyond all the science and chemistry, what matters most is how you individually tolerate them.

But, for now, trust me: You don't need any of this and you will do much, much better by simply sticking to high-quality animal foods 99% of the time. Embracing high-quality animal foods — and consuming only the best of the best — will be the fastest and easiest way to make real progress on the journey to optimal health.

Chapter Seven

Food Quality: The Biggest Factor in Nutrition and Health

Every day, countless new articles, TV reports, YouTube videos, and research studies talk about one food or another being "healthy" for you. No doubt, some foods are generally better. And others are always bad. But labeling any specific thing as unquestionably "healthy" misses the biggest factor in nutrition and human health.

Food quality is KING! What the animal was raised on determines its vitamin, mineral, and overall nutritional content. This means that you always want to consume animals that themselves ate their natural diet.

Cows should be eating grass. Pigs should be foraging for leaves, roots, and bugs. If they instead spend their lives eating low-quality and unnatural industrial feed, they will have fewer nutrients in their muscles, fat, and organs.

A steak is not just a steak. An egg is not just an egg. Salmon is not just salmon. Milk is not just milk. Bacon, from the right animal that lived the right way, can be very healthy and nutritious. Or, as most varieties are, it can be highly processed crap full of Omega-6 fatty acids, preservatives, and commercial poison. Garbage in, garbage out. Pretty simple.

The Vital Importance of Food Quality

How much difference can there really be between grass-fed and grain-fed beef? It's a reasonable question that many people don't fully grasp. It doesn't help that the marketing around grass-fed beef generally promotes it as an organic product that is free from "contaminants" (including steroids, hormones, and antibiotics) and more humane.

Make no mistake: There is a definite benefit to not ingesting those industrial compounds. But there has unfortunately been little done to raise awareness about the nutritional differences, and this is what is really fundamental to the Ancestral Indigenous Diet.

The nutrient difference can be drastic. A conventionally raised grain-fed ribeye or New York strip, honestly, gives you almost no fat-soluble vitamins. You will get a few of the commonly obtained B Vitamins and some minerals. But, by comparison, some grass-fed bone marrow will effectively give you all the nutrition you need for the entire day.

You should also know that different foods are affected by feedlot production in different ways. Pork and chicken are impacted by industrial feed more than beef because of how the digestive systems of ruminant animals work. In particular, it alters the Omega ratio in the animal's fat, among other factors. Many people report feeling great on grain-fed steak but become more lethargic, or just feel "off" if they eat too much conventionally raised pork. The differences in how the different animals react to grain feeding is a big reason why.

This isn't an invitation to eat feedlot beef. It's not good for you! But it means that, in a pinch, eating a steak at Applebees once in awhile may not affect you as negatively as eating conventional pork chops every day.

Beyond the barnyard, we see differences in the ocean as well. Wild-caught fish, especially salmon, has an excellent nutrient profile that is much better than farmed varieties. No matter what the fish ate or where it was raised, there will still be a pollution consideration that can be worrisome to some degree. Fish is something of a double-edged sword.

Then again, especially for those of us eating in North America, wild-caught fish typically have the benefit of maintaining some year-round consistency. Sure, you may be worried about the potential pollution factor even with wild-caught fish. But a piece of Pacific sockeye salmon, by and large, will usually have a good nutrient profile regardless of when it was caught. And a fish pulled aboard a ship during high season then flash frozen will store its nutrients well until it reaches your plate.

We don't always see this with grass-fed beef. When the cow is coming off summer pasture, it is always packed with nutrients. But these same cows often eat hay during the winter. Even though hay is close to their natural, preferred food source — and way better than industrial soy or corn feed covered in the herbicide atrazine — it doesn't allow the cows to store as many vitamins. Then there is Vitamin D to think about. The winter season means the cows won't see enough sun to convert high levels of Vitamin D3. This is one reason why we see indigenous groups fermenting or preserving foods from the late summer and fall.

In short, even grass-fed beef isn't always grass-fed beef. There will be nutrient differences depending upon the time of year, where it's from, and the grass it ate.

Major Differences in Food Quality

In animal foods, we are primarily concerned with vitamins. For plants, because they don't contain bioavailable vitamins in considerable amounts, it's minerals. As noted, the ultimate vitamin content in the beef products we consume depends not just on the cow's feed but on the season it was slaughtered and even the actual quality of the pasture and soil.

Such factors are very difficult to know. It's one thing to buy a plastic-wrapped package that says "grass-fed" at Whole Foods and another to find a trustworthy specialty supplier that guarantees "grass-fed" *and* "grass-finished" beef. Then it is another thing altogether to actually know your local farmer personally and have visited the farm and pasture to see where the cows are raised, fed, and slaughtered.

I get it: This is asking a lot. Do we really have to go through all this just to eat dinner? Besides, can I really even tell the difference? Could I actually pick out the more nutritious steak if two very different options were placed in front of me — let alone have an idea what type of pasture is optimal for a cow?

In some sense, you probably can't as an untrained consumer. It would be great if we had better nutritional facts to rely on. This would help everybody learn the difference between grass-fed and grain-fed beef generally. (Side note: Doing this type of testing is a personal goal of mine. It is expensive and so far hasn't generated that much demand from the marketplace. But I hope to help provide more clarity on this information in the future.)

All that said, there are ways for a trained eye to spot food quality. And you will get better at it in time if you learn the signs.

How do you tell? For one, the meat from grass-fed and older animals is generally darker. The fat should also be beige, or even bordering on yellow, not stark white.

Even better than training your eye, you should educate your tongue. It is far easier to identify properly raised animals by taste. Because if they are not raised right, the fat will have a hard texture and something of an off, acrid taste.

Assessing fish is generally less of an issue since it is usually labeled "wild-caught" or "farm-raised" at the fishmonger. Although wild-caught fish, especially shellfish, is a very reliable source of certain nutrients, as a rule, farmed fish can be problematic due to pollution concerns. In general, it still is usually better — in most cases — than feedlot-raised beef, pork, and chicken. But some people react very badly to the toxins and other negative substances they contain

I personally feel like death if I eat more than a small amount of farmed salmon. So if that is the only thing available, I just avoid it altogether and rely on brains, shellfish, eggs, cod liver fish oil pills, cod liver, or another good source for Omega-3s.

Eating Local: Not Just for Hipsters

My standards for food quality are ridiculously high. In both my personal life and my business as a food distributor, I go to stupid lengths to find the very best. This means I have spent countless hours searching around my local area for the top options — and it certainly helps in some ways that I live in New York City. There are just a ton of options in the nation's largest metro area and I try to take advantage of them all.

Then again, some people living in a small town in Montana may have even better luck by just driving 10 miles down the road. You may be able to ask a rancher for 20 pounds of grass-fed veal liver and be set for the whole season — though good luck finding salmon roe or fresh crab consistently in a landlocked town of 5,000 people.

Wherever you are, there are probably some tradeoffs. First of all, don't instantly fall for the marketing hype. Local *does not* necessarily mean quality. They farm 30 miles away may not be a multinational that buys agrochemicals by the cargo ship. But you can't always trust everything they say. And even the ones with the goods tend to rip people off. I have learned this firsthand — and way too many times. You need to be careful.

Then there are other factors. Conventionally raised beef may be cheaper in Texas and Colorado, whereas Massachusetts and Vermont have a farmer's market culture that promotes CSA (Community Supported Agriculture) options for pastured pork or raw milk. These places also have cheaper seafood. But long winters mean any beef you get in February wasn't recently feeding off grass, as it may have been at certain Texas farms all year round.

Getting the best food quality at the best price is about understanding what is available. Do your best to find food locally and learn what you can buy online or in retail stores as more of a commodity (like canned cod liver or cod liver oil). In the winter, it may make sense to lean on stuff like this to make sure you get your nutrients and consume steak more so for calorie and protein needs.

You Get What You Pay For

This may all sound great. But what if you can't afford grass-fed meat? Getting all the nutrients you need — and avoiding inflammation — really is the most important aspect of your health. So it is something you need to start prioritizing in your life. This may take some sacrifices. Everything worth achieving usually does and this is no exception.

Look, everyone has their own definition of a budget. Some people really do lack the means to afford the type of animal products they should be consuming. That is a sad statement on the job market and how most people eat in this country.

Still, there is a huge difference between feeling like you have to live off of potatoes, rice, and ramen vs. being strict about your spending and finding a way to be healthy. And this isn't like paying for a gym membership. You always have the option to spend either $100 per month or $0 per month on a gym membership. But nobody can spend $0 on food. You will be paying *something* to eat. The question is more about *how* you spend your money.

The average person in the United States spends $660 per month on food, according to the most recent statistics from the U.S. Bureau of Labor Statistics (BLS). This is even higher for many people living in cities like Seattle ($913), San Diego ($832), Houston ($762), and Los Angeles ($727).

You may think that sounds like a ton of money. But we're not just talking about groceries here. This includes all spending: that daily breakfast bagel, going out to lunch twice a week, and treating yourself to an ice cream at the end of a hard week.

Of the $7,923 spent on food by the average American in 2018, nearly half — $3,459, or 43% — came on "food away from home." While nobody is suggesting you can never eat out, we all know that our money goes a lot farther at the grocery store — even if you go shopping at "Whole Paycheck" or the farmer's market.

So ask yourself this: Is higher-quality food something you truly can't afford? Or is it something that you just care about less than new clothes, football tickets, or video games?

Food Quality on a Budget

Some people really are scraping by and can't come up with anywhere near $150 per week for food. Others in the same boat might be trying to improve their health on a college student budget.

At the end of the day, yeah, there are ways to make a carnivore diet work on a few dollars a day. This mostly means you'll be buying conventionally raised ground beef, off-the-shelf grocery store eggs, and regular old butter. This is super cheap stuff. Generally, the best solution isn't to start purchasing a lot of cheap, grain-fed meat. It's to go for more affordable wild-caught fish, like mackerel and herring.

You may even consider possibly substituting in foods like rice or potatoes for the remainder of your calories. This is a big sacrifice, but you will avoid the troubling agrochemicals that are rampant in conventional beef feed. A diet of 50% wild fish and 50% sweet potatoes is infinitely better than a feedlot beef diet.

Ultimately, the nutritional differences between grain-fed and grass-fed beef can be made up in other ways. But the agrochemicals — especially the estrogenic herbicide atrazine used widely in soy and corn feed — cause hormonal issues. This can be especially damaging for male fertility, according to some studies. So, in many respects, you need to try to avoid the bad stuff as much as you look to obtain beneficial nutrition.

At this price, you are really losing a lot of the health benefits and not getting all the nutrition you need. It is still better than the Standard American Diet — especially for reducing inflammation — and even commercial eggs have more nutrition than a lot of the "health food" people waste their money on. But there will be a tradeoff. High-quality food, unfortunately, does come at something of a premium.

Another good way to reduce costs is with supplements. Getting DHA and Vitamin A through actual animal sources will always be better, but there are decent fish oil pills, cod liver oil, Vitamin K2, and Vitamin D3 supplements on the market at reasonable prices.

If you can't find the money for eggs from pastured chickens or raw cheese, there may be compromises worth making on occasion. Supermarket eggs should be avoided, but organic Omega-3 eggs are passable. So eating (slightly) more conventional versions of these foods and supplementing with Vitamin K2 can be something of a solution to make sure you don't become deficient. Fish oil alone — especially from the cheaper pills — likely won't give you all the Omega-3s or Vitamin A that you really need in your diet. But it could help until you can make a little more money to buy wild-caught fish more often.

There are also sardines, canned salmon, and canned cod liver. Depending upon the brand, these are not always the highest quality. But everyone can afford these options though, and consuming them even once or twice per week is better than nothing. You really can improve your nutrition without spending $50 per day on grass-fed Wagyu beef and Copper River salmon.

In the long run, finding the money for better food will pay off. Think of it as an investment. I'm a big believer in spending as much as you can on better food.

Even in just a few months, you will become much closer to the optimal version of yourself. You will have more energy. You will feel better. And this is exactly what you need to find more success in all aspects of your life. With a little luck, a better version of yourself may just be able to start earning enough money to buy even better food.

Eating Nose to Tail

There is one other big factor in nutrition that is constantly overlooked. Eating the entire animal — something commonly referred to as eating "nose to tail" for land animals — will give complete nutrition. This means you will get everything your body needs and in natural ratios.

This is because animals store the nutrients we need all throughout their body. Muscle meat (and, really, only a few specific cuts) is what most modern diners prefer. But cows don't store that many nutrients in their muscles. There are a few vitamins and lots of protein, but not much else. So you can't just eat a few steaks and expect to get everything you need — unless maybe you found some mutated Wagyu steak raised on the highest-quality pasture in the world. You've gotta eat the fat and the organs too if you want to get the actual nutrition.

The same thing applies to clams, mussels, and crabs. They all offer complete nutrition as well. And you actually do get all of those nutrients because they are small animals that you essentially eat whole. This doesn't necessarily make them better. But it does mean that seafood makes it easier for you. Everything is right there in just a few bites. Obtaining their full nutritional profile is as easy as ordering one for your plate. Going to a restaurant and slugging down half a dozen oysters with some lemon juice is about the healthiest thing you can do.

And that's just the way it will always be — at least until we figure out how to shrink a cow down to the size of an egg so we can get it all in one bite. Without that technology, you will just have to learn to enjoy some organs and eat fattier meat.

If that doesn't sound appetizing, you can cheat a little bit. You can also get this complete nutrient profile through animal products such as dairy and eggs. Like a clam, both of these products contain all the essential substances your body needs. And this is why I advocate for raw, grass-fed dairy so much. It's delicious and far more approachable than a raw oyster.

Along with food quality and complete nutrition, we should be considering the specific nutrient profile of each item we consume. As you learn more about all the different foods that will become important in your diet, you will start to understand this all better. That way, you will know how often you need to eat foods high in, for example, DHA or Vitamin K2 to reinforce your daily effort to eat products that offer complete nutrition on their own.

Chapter Eight

Food Sourcing:
What to Eat and How to Get It

When it comes to food quality, there is good news and there is bad news. The good news is that there is great food out there that will give you all the nutrients you ever need. The bad news is that it can be hard to get your hands on. And even if you do find the very best, it can be expensive.

This is simply the world we live in, especially in the United States. Corporate food producers have spent decades chasing profits and pushing volume over quality. And consumers have gone along for the ride because price and convenience win out over everything in this day and age.

The sad reality is that if you want to be healthy and get all the nutrients you need, you do need to start putting some effort into "food sourcing." The more time and effort you devote to it, the better the results will be. You will get as much out of this as you put in.

For some people, the biggest change is a mindset shift. Every year, more "specialty" animal products go mainstream and become more widely available. There is now a larger market for organic and local food than at any time since your grandparents were growing up. (Back then, almost all the food was high-quality food. So much for modern progress.)

Maybe your local grocery store has great grass-fed steaks that you can even afford, but you simply have been buying conventionally raised beef out of habit. Now that you understand the reasons to buy grass-fed instead, it's just a matter of doing it.

Other people may have to start going to a different store. Costco frozen hamburger patties are out. Whole Foods grass-fed strip steaks are in. Even going from the cheapest butter in the store to Kerrygold is a step in the right direction. And don't overlook local Asian markets, fish markets, or wholesale distributors. These spots may not have been on your radar before. But they are all over the place and can be great sources for great food — at great prices — if you live near a large population center.

Making the Effort: Levels of Food Sourcing

Knowing that you have to look harder for better food is half the battle. But that won't win you the war. To achieve your optimal health and to really follow the Ancestral Indigenous Diet, you will probably need to try a bit harder than simply going to Whole Foods.

This is a decent start, but the quality is all over the map and it becomes quite expensive quite quickly. Because, unfortunately, even if you think you are buying the best quality meat, misleading marketing terms have allowed companies to sell feedlot meat as "organic" and even "grass fed." Both organic soy and corn stalks fall under those constituents.

This doesn't have to become an obsession (like it has for me). It may be very easy to find a local farm that raises grass-fed beef — without hormones or antibiotics — and will sell you pounds of liver all year long. Maybe you can just drive a half-hour out to the farm once a month for a massive haul of steak, beef fat, liver, eggs, and cheese. BOOM. You've solved all your food sourcing issues in about the same amount of time that you spend getting haircuts each month. Some farms even deliver.

But it probably won't be that easy. And just when you find the best source of liver ever, the season will change and you'll be coming up dry. The raw milk provider you relied on for months might go out of business. The fishmonger that has the best fish roe may stop stocking it.

For those problems — and especially for people just getting started — the following guidelines will help you get going. These four basic levels of food sourcing offer something of a roadmap that you can follow as you continue to get more advanced.

Level 1: Beginner

Sources: Supermarkets, wholesale retail locations (like Costco), Asian markets for fish (like H Mart)

Pros/Cons: Food access is limited, pricing and quality is hit or miss

Level 2: Moderate

Sources: Farms, farmers markets, co-ops, local butchers

Pros/Cons: Better quality, more expensive, meat is often frozen

Level 3: Advanced

Sources: Restaurant purveyors, buying whole primal cuts

Pros/Cons: High cost, may need business license/credit line, having personal meat storage for bulk

Level 4: Expert

Sources: Buying whole animals for slaughter, hunting, owning a farm

Pros/Cons: best food possible, very intensive in terms of time, effort, and knowledge

How Much Does It Cost?

There are great bargains all over. And some of the best foods out there really aren't that expensive. Still, in a general sense, you will largely get what you pay for. There are ways to get most of your nutrients on a budget, but one goal in your food sourcing should be to spend more on higher-quality products.

How much can you really get at different levels? The following offers a rough guideline of what you can expect to find at various price points.

Conventional Diet: $150 per month

Core Foods: Cheap wild fish, whatever meat you can afford, conventional eggs, cheap dairy, canned fish, supplements, substituting in some cheaper plant foods

Middle of the Road: $300-$400 per month

Core Foods: Basic steaks, grass-fed organs, cheaper wild-caught fish

Perfect Diet: $600+ per month

Core Foods: Grass-fed everything, pastured pork, true free-range eggs, raw dairy, wild-caught fish eggs, wild game, trustworthy cod liver oil

Prized Foods

Say you've struck it rich. Congrats. You now have all the money in the world and access to every animal on every farm. In an ideal world, what must you start eating to get all the nutrients you need and stay free of inflammation?

First of all, don't always think about this in terms of cost. Some of the best foods are going to cost a bit more. But prized foods aren't necessarily expensive. A fish-monger fileting fish tends to throw out the eggs and organs. You can even get them for free sometimes.

Throughout history, our ancestral forebearers have shown preferences for certain foods. For the indigenous hunter who we want to follow, the preference would have been the fattier parts of wild game such as the marrow or kidney fat. The same goes for animals living in the wild. For a bear, it might be the skin, brains, and eggs of a salmon swimming upstream. The one consistent factor is a craving for calorically dense nutrition. If we cannot obtain all the nutrients *and* all the energy we need, we wouldn't be able to survive times of famine.

Today, of course, finding calories is never a problem. Our issue is acquiring the micronutrients we need without all the garbage that causes inflammation and many modern diseases.

Ancestral food preferences can also be seen in the wide variety of preparation methods that indigenous groups used. Different parts of each animal would be prepared differently.

If a hunter killed a caribou, for example, the group might have enjoyed the lower leg bone marrow raw then boiled the upper leg marrow. Maybe they boil the head to get at the brains and then roast the kidney fat over a fire as it dries out. One tribe may have given the raw salmon eggs they found inside the catch to their nursing women. Another may have added it to seal-meat soup.

In many recorded accounts, it seems the preference was to first eat nutrient-dense foods, including fat, whenever calories were otherwise plentiful and there wasn't a major threat of starvation.

In the 1937 book *Foods America Gave the World*, A. Hyatt Verrill wrote about one tradition of eating honey ants he encountered. "In many places," he wrote, "the natives are very fond of the female of queen ants when filled with roe … In Mexico no wedding breakfast is considered complete without a side dish of the big honey ants."

He found that, in Barbados and other areas of the Caribbean, the natives consider "sea eggs" — a spiny sea urchin that in "certain seasons is full of roe" — to be "by far the best of the seafoods." And in other places, "the eggs of the iguanas are also highly esteemed by the natives."

Today, when I eat for nutrient density, I am generally looking for high-value foods like liver (for all vitamins and especially its unmatched Vitamin A content), salmon roe or other fish eggs (for DHA and EPA), bone marrow (for complete nutrition), and brain (for DHA and vitamins general).

These were prized in ancient times as well, but in reality, almost every single part of an animal besides the muscle meat was coveted. Kidney, sweetbreads, spleen, thymus, and reproductive organs. They all serve a purpose in acquiring both nutrition and calories.

The Top Ancestral Indigenous Diet Prized Foods

- Beef/Veal Liver (All Vitamins and Minerals, Copper/Vitamin A/B Vitamins notably high)
- Brains (DHA, EPA, Vitamin C, Vitamin E)
- Kidneys (All Vitamins and Minerals, Selenium notably high)
- Bone Marrow (Fat Soluble Vitamins, Calorically Dense)
- Salmon/Fish Roe (All Vitamins and Minerals, DHA/Iodine notably high)
- Cod Liver/Cod Liver Oil (Similar to liver but has high omega 3 and iodine)
- Shellfish (All Vitamins and Minerals, Oysters high B Vitamins, varies depending on item)
- Wild-Caught Fish (complete nutrition if guts are eaten)
- Raw Summer/Fall Dairy (All Fat Soluble Vitamins, Minerals besides Iron)
- Eggs (Complete Balanced Nutrition)

Meat: Beef, Poultry, Pork, and More

The Ancestral Indigenous Diet is a carnivore diet. Fat and meat will be your primary focus after the nutrient-dense organs, roe, and other prized items. What you should always be looking for are low Omega-6 meats. Grass-fed and pastured animals are always better in this regard and should be your top choice. If you want to be strict and eat optimally, they should be your only choice.

But if you do have to buy conventionally raised meat — due to price or local availability — it is better to stick to beef or lamb. Even when raised on soy and corn feed, they will have a better Omega-3 to Omega-6 ratio.

As for specific cuts that should be praised, fattier cuts like belly, brisket, and short-rib don't require additional fat to be added to the meal. Then, as the cuts get leaner, they would have been less conducive to survival and nutrient density. The classic ribeye and New York strip are always good options for us today, especially if you can get the butcher to include a generous fat cap.

Pork and chicken unfortunately are drastically higher in Omega-6 because of how their digestive system is affected by grain feeding. For this reason, most people who eat a carnivore diet stick mostly to beef. Unfortunately, soy-free pasture-raised chicken is much more expensive than grass-fed beef. Not only that, it's incredibly difficult to find without buying whole animals from local farms.

And remember: Just because it's labeled "pasture raised" doesn't mean it wasn't fed 70% corn. If you're finding it in your local grocery, chances are it isn't what it says on the package. Governmental regulation for all these terms are shockingly loose. Be wary of what you are buying, and know that color is a great indicator of meat quality, especially pork or chicken. Pork should be red like beef, and pasture-raised chicken will be much darker than the glowing white meat you're used to seeing.

Ancestral Indigenous Diet Meats

- Fatty Cuts (Belly, Shortribs, Brisket, Chuck Roast) of Grass-fed/Pastured Animals (general nutrition, protein, calories)
- Other Cuts of Grass-fed/Pastured Animals (general nutrition, protein, calories)

Eggs and Dairy

Eggs and dairy are double-edged swords. At the highest level of quality, they are incredible sources of nutrition. On the other hand, the typical stuff you find in the store is usually very poor and there are overarching allergy concerns for many people. Honestly, it's bad enough that the typical versions are generally not fit to consume.

Eggs, in particular, suffer the same high Omega-6 problem that pork and chicken do, although all eggs do have substantial Vitamin K2 and Omega-3 content not found in grocery store pigs and poultry. But as with chicken and pork, the "pasture raised" or "free range" label is not an indicator of quality. You honestly never know what you're really getting from brand-name eggs. When I purchase eggs, I make sure to buy them from a local farmer that I can guarantee does not use soy in the feed. It's the only way to know what is actually in the box and ensures you get a lower Omega-6 intake and a higher nutrient content.

Supermarket dairy is even worse than supermarket eggs. It is pasteurized, homogenized, rancid (oxidized), and devoid of almost all the nutrition it should have. Even the "grass-fed" butter in stores, like Kerrygold, is far from what we should be consuming. Kerrygold products may be better than conventional — and an option for some people — but they are not ideal.

Real, raw, grass-fed dairy products, on the other hand, are nutritionally complete and provide some amount of all the nutrients you need. Whether it's milk, butter, cream, or cheese, it will have every single vitamin and mineral — plus it's just a delicious, approachable food. It even has other beneficial compounds, including bacteria for our microbiome and enzymes that aid in digestion.

One downside is that allergies and intolerances are abundant. Switching from A1 protein milk to A2 protein milk may help some people. Goat and sheep milk are naturally A2 varieties (which have smaller fat molecules and are easier to digest). But they can be prohibitively expensive for day-to-day use. Raw goat milk may be manageable at around $15 per gallon (compared to $10 for raw cow milk). But raw sheep milk can cost upwards of $30-$40 per gallon and it comes with more than double the calories.

Unlike eggs, you can't really go for the conventional variety at all. Grocery-store, pasteurized milk gives you next to no benefits. If dairy is consumed, it's hard to justify anything outside of raw, grass-fed. Cheese can be a decent option if you can't find a local farm with raw products. Various imported varieties, like Parmigiano-Reggiano from Italy, are protected products and always made from unpasteurized milk. This means it will always have some good nutrients, and Whole Foods also often carries aged, raw, grass-fed cheese from local products that are priced reasonably. Even many supermarkets have raw cheese if you know what to look for.

Top Ancestral Indigenous Diet Egg & Dairy Options

- Farm, Soy-Free Eggs (All Fat Soluble Vitamins, Minerals, Fatty Acids)
- Raw Summer Dairy (All Fat Soluble Vitamins, Minerals besides Iron)

Fish and Seafood

Fish is in the same boat as eggs and dairy. The good stuff is great. The bad is very bad. In fact, most farmed fish could arguably be considered one of the least healthy foods we can consume because of the crazy levels of toxins and pollutants introduced by certain fishing practices.

On the other hand, wild-caught fish — especially shellfish, mollusks, and fatty fish — are literally the healthiest foods we can eat. High-quality fish can replace meat, eggs, and dairy in your diet. There are many indigenous and native peoples who consumed fish as virtually their only source of protein — (although they usually needed another source of energy from plant foods because most fish isn't abundant in fat and calories). First Nation Alaskans, for example, would dip their fish in seal oil to increase the caloric content.

In all cases, live fish is best (especially shellfish), followed by fresh fatty fish (like Pacific salmon), then frozen (like salmon or mackerel), and then canned (various). But no matter the state it's in when you buy it, it always has to be wild-caught. There are a few acceptable exceptions of farmed fish that are fed a wild diet (like oysters and mussels) but you should still always be careful.

Top Ancestral Indigenous Diet Seafood Options

- Oysters (All Vitamins and Minerals, High B12 and Omega 3)
- Fatty Shellfish Crab/Lobster (All Vitamins and Minerals)
- Other Shellfish / Mussels (All Vitamins and Minerals, may be low if lean)
- Wild-Caught Fatty Fish (All Vitamins and Minerals, High Omega 3)

Fermented Foods

Fermented foods — or rotten foods — have been a staple of human civilization since time immemorial. Even people today often eat old food all day without even realizing it. Yogurt for breakfast, ham and cheese on sourdough for lunch, and an aged steak for dinner.

These are all months old and seen as delicious. But tell someone you're eating certain other fermented foods in cultures and watch them get grossed out immediately. This is mostly because it's not what we've grown up with — although the smell can certainly be a turn off.

Every indigenous group ate fermented food in a variety of ways. Some let meat rot in the African sun for a week. People in Alaska might leave it under a log in near-freezing temperatures for a year. Whether they knew what they were doing or not, letting the food rot gave it beneficial bacteria and altered its vitamin content.

There are beneficial microbes that grow when meat ferments in a certain way, and these bacteria also increase the Vitamin K2 content of the food, something that is very important for skeletal development. This Vitamin K2 content is the main nutrient we are looking for when it comes to fermented foods, although the bacteria has its own benefits for our gut and immune system.

These days, we call this "high meat," a term taken from certain native people. And this stuff reeks. I mean it. I've made jars of high meat, and it is putrid. It doesn't really belong in a house.

When looking at the bacteria that form, there are several important categories: Native Healthy Microbes, Native Unhealthy Microbes, and Opportunistic Environmental Bacteria. What turns rotten meat into something potentially beneficial is an environment where the healthy microbes can thrive unaltered. There are so many ways indigenous people made high meat, but after a few months, it becomes something you could almost compare to a nice cheese.

This really isn't something anyone should be doing at home. You can just eat some actual cheese like a normal human being. While it won't be exactly the same as eating old, gross meat, some raw, grass-fed cheese will give you the Vitamin K2 you need in its MK4 animal form. And your friends, family, and significant others are less likely to call you insane.

Top Ancestral Indigenous Diet Fermented Options

- Raw, Grass-Fed Cheese (Vitamin K2)
- High Meat (Vitamin K2)

I Have to Eat What?!??!

I have some great news for you: We are not actually living in 40,000 BC and we don't necessarily have to be eating rotten animal fat, raw lamb brains, or whole goat eyeballs to get by. I personally have tried all the wacky and weird things you could imagine. And I will continue eating brains, testicles, and other organs most people wouldn't even touch. But that's just me. What can ya do?

Funny story: The closest I came to dying was probably when I tried to swallow an eyeball whole. I figured, this way, I could get all the nutritional benefits without actually having to taste the thing. It was a great plan — until it got caught in my windpipe. After about 30 seconds of thinking, "Is this really how Frank Boy is going to die?" it popped out of my mouth. Lesson learned. I now thoroughly chew everything I eat — even if it tastes like eyeballs.

The Ancestral Indigenous Diet starts with a micronutrient priority. Get those vitamins and minerals in. You probably do need to eat some liver for Vitamin A. (It's the only high-volume source unless you're sucking down half a gallon of summer milk.) And salmon roe really can't be beat for Omega-3s. (Although some salmon every week is fine.)

Once you have your Vitamin A, DHA, Vitamin K2, and Vitamin D3 accounted for, you can start moving down the list to the other main nutrients. After that, the goal is to get the proteins and fats you need. But we're now starting to talk about meeting calorie and energy needs. The goal here is to get as much as you need without overeating (we still don't want to get chubby) or promoting any inflammatory response.

Keep Getting Denser

To actually follow the Ancestral Indigenous Diet, you need to understand the importance of food quality. You will never achieve the nutrient density you need unless you get all the vitamins and minerals you need while cutting out all the low-quality foods that cause inflammation and other problems. And as we've learned, food quality and food sourcing are inherently linked. To get one, you need to get good at the other.

That said, this diet is different from many popular all-of-nothing eating trends. With the Keto Diet, you're either in ketosis or you're not. With Paleo or something like Whole 30, you're either sticking to the approved food list or your not. The same even goes for Veganism, as horrible as that life choice is for your health, and Intermittent Fasting, which requires certain time intervals to be met.

I am definitely not suggesting that you only go halfway with my diet. You will get much better results and be much healthier if you strictly follow all the advice I am offering.

But you will also see benefits just by making the changes you can make right this moment. As you learn more about the different nutrients available in different foods — like how to get all the DHA you need without spending much — you will have no excuses. This book offers the basics you need, and my YouTube channel contains even more nuanced information on all sorts of topics related to food and health.

Keep learning more and more. You will find out that off-cuts of lamb or beef can be found at a price you can afford, for example. You should keep making sacrifices in other areas of your life so you can afford to eat better quality foods, including grass-fed beef. You can find different types of fish eggs available at the local Asian market that you had never even heard of (like monkfish, which isn't a bad option). And, hopefully, in time, you will earn more money and certain things may become more feasible to buy.

Food sourcing is a journey. It is not something you will perfect overnight. Even after devoting so much time to this over the past decade, I have still been ripped off or wound up receiving farmed salmon that the purveyor promised was wild caught. It happens.

But even small changes will help at the beginning. Eating liver once a week and getting a decent cod liver oil supplement will instantly put key nutrients in your diet that you have probably been lacking for years. As you get more advanced and learn how different foods affect your stomach, mental clarity, and mood, you will only get better. You will begin to know what to buy and which expensive products simply don't seem worth the money to you. You will figure out whether it's even worth your time to find raw dairy or if those "farm-fresh" eggs are the real deal.

Make no mistake: I recommend jumping straight into the deep-end and radically changing how you eat. Get the best food you can and don't be too worried about the initial price. You will be much better off for it and you will figure out how to cut costs without cutting quality in months two, three, and four. But if you do have to ease your way into the pool, you will still be much better off than you were just last week.

The most important practical information is to increase the amount of quality animal foods you are eating. It's better to have oysters with cookies than cake and cookies.

Chapter Nine

Food Preparation: Cooking and Eating to Maximize Nutrition

I have already told you about my former life in the gym as a bodybuilder and many people already know me as a nutrition advocate on YouTube. But you might not know that much of my professional experience lies in New York City restaurants, working as both a bartender and waiter.

That is where Frankie Boy learned pretty much everything he knows about the culinary arts. I really did pick up so much along the way. It's amazing what you see in some of these kitchens and steakhouses about how to prepare and perfect certain dishes. I'm a humble guy. But on top of my passion for learning about food from a nutrition standpoint, I like to consider myself as a pretty good cook.

I even made it on MasterChef to audition a few years back. My time there was unfortunately cut quite short, and the quick version is that I wasn't exactly at my best during my appearance on the show. But I still think Frankie The Chef could stack up against the best of 'em if ever given another shot.

That's another story though. (As is my brief stint working for internet legend Salt Bae when he launched his New York restaurant.) For now, I only mention it so you know I'm not just some filthy caveman who only spends his days gnawing on raw liver, sheep brains, and fish eggs then washing it down with a bloody Mary — made with actual blood.

I know what actual cuisine is, and I pride myself on my culinary knowledge. Just because I have limited my diet down to mostly the essentials — choosing most days to grill grass-fed steaks seasoned only with salt and a side of fresh organs — doesn't mean I don't appreciate great food.

But there is a big difference between how we *should* eat and how we *do* eat. And as discussed earlier when it comes to traditional grain preparation methods, there is a right way — and a wrong way — to do things if you want to cook for optimal nutrition.

The good news is that this isn't exactly rocket science. There's no need to break this all down into an instruction manual or cookbook. But I wanted to take a little bit of time here to clear up a few common misconceptions about how cooking affects nutrition and offer some handy preparation tips for any novices out there. Even you long-time grill-masters still have room to learn.

The following won't give you a complete understanding of how to cook and eat food on the Ancestral Indigenous Diet. But these are some good starting guidelines that you can build on for the rest of your life. That way, you will have a diet that satisfies you in all ways, from nutrient density and culinary exploration to enjoying real flavor and getting that perfect sear.

Carnivore Cooking 101

The most common cooking methods you should get acquainted with are grilling, pan searing, and baking in an oven. Indigenous people would have done their own versions of these techniques as well as boiling, steaming, smoking, drying, pulverizing, and rendering fats.

To be sure, there really isn't any wrong way to cook your meat. Different methods can affect the nutrient profile, but a lot of that will come down to raw vs. cooked. But before we get to all that, let's just talk about a few simple aspects of cooking that will help you enjoy your meat a bit more.

Frankie Boy's Signature Style

I cook almost every meal over a wood fire. What can I say? I'm just a sucker for the classics. Nothing tastes better. It's also easier and doesn't make a mess all over my stove.

I do, however, use a bit of an unconventional technique. Some people will tell you charcoal is the holy grail for grilling. But it takes forever to heat up. That just isn't practical on a day-to-day basis when you're always eating meat.

On the other extreme is gas. Sure, some pitmaster from Texas might say propane grills are an embarrassment and unfit for real meat lovers. Chill out though, guys. You can't beat propane for convenience, and we all have a life to live.

To get something like the best of both worlds — primal nature meets modern ingenuity — Frankie Boy found some middle ground. I use a small, cheap gas-start propane grill that I've modified a bit to take seasoned firewood as well.

I did it by taking an old grate and putting it on the bottom next to the burner where the flames come out. So I get the gas going then toss some small pieces of wood on there. This means it gets going fast and I still get some extra flavor and smoke from the kindling. For me, this is the only way to go anymore. Even in New York, I get out there in the snow. It's that good.

But I understand grilling every day isn't for everyone. So you will want to have a good cast iron or carbon steel pan to sear your meat on the stovetop for those occasions. Roasting or baking is also good for certain types of meat, so you'll want a few baking sheets and racks.

The Searing Secret

Everyone always talks about moist meat and not letting your steak, pork, chicken, or turkey dry out. It's the cardinal sin of cooking! Perhaps that's why so many people misunderstand one important part about cooking meat: You don't just want — you *need* — a dry surface. Yes, you want the final product to be moist — but that's on the inside.

To start the cooking, though, it is absolutely essential to dry off the surface on the outside. This is what helps get such a great, flavorful crust on a steak (but also every other type of meat). Otherwise, if the surface is wet, you end up just steaming the outside rather than getting that hard, brown sear that brings a cut to the next level.

The best bet is to leave it in the fridge on a rack or towels overnight. Then use paper towels to pat it very, very dry right before you get ready to put it into the cast iron or on the grill. If you want to go the extra mile, you can add salt the day before to further harden the exterior but opinions vary on when is the best time to salt a steak when it comes to flavor.

Adequate Heat

When pan searing, you need to find the Goldilocks temperature. If the pan isn't hot enough, you won't get a crust. If it's too hot, however, you get a burnt crust before the interior has time to cook at all. And to make matters even more complicated, this temperature differs depending upon the dish. You'll want to cook a rare ribeye hot and fast while crispy-skin salmon filet needs a softer touch and more time in the pan.

Especially with a steak, make sure to frequently move the meat around the cooking surface for even heat distribution. Use tongs to get all four sides and don't forget about the ends. Chicken is more forgiving in general and can be tossed around as necessary to get some brown flavor all over. Salmon should sit still, skin side down, for almost the entire cooking process until you flip it over for the final minute to finish it through.

Cooking Temperatures

If you want a specific doneness, having an instant read thermometer is very helpful. You will get better at this in time, but having one handy will help you figure out how you like your meat and get used to your stove and equipment.

I personally eat my steak blue-rare. But from a culinary perspective, 120-123 degrees Farenheit is rare, 124-127 degrees is medium rare, and 130 degrees is medium. Anything past that is well done — and probably best left for the dogs. For chicken you generally want to shoot for 150F for white meat and 175 degrees for dark meat. For pork, I try to go to 135 degrees, although some food safety pros would probably suggest going higher than that (at around 145 degrees).

And don't forget about resting time and "carryover cooking time." To get your meat to settle in at a desired temperature, you need to take it off the heat about 5-10 degrees before its at the mark. That way, once you remove it from the heating element and set it aside to rest, it will continue to cook for another few minutes and hit the temp.

Adequate Fat

Aside from baking and smoking, in most other cases, meat needs some fat to cook properly. This is what helps distribute the heat and caramelize the crust. Without sufficient fat, honestly it's usually impossible to get a proper crust.

This is generally no problem for a fatty ribeye or good old ground beef patty. But you will want to use some external fat when dealing with a lean piece of meat. In a cast iron or other pan, this can be done by starting with a bit of fat (whether animal fat like tallow, butter, or ghee for its high smoke point).

Or on the grill, you will want to baste it while it cooks. And don't be scared to lather on the butter lavishly. I go with clarified butter or tallow usually, and it not only gets the grates well oiled but gets the fire going better. Be careful about flare ups. You don't want to set the house on fire, but a few flames jumping up into the meat will only add that flavor you are trying so hard to get on the meat in the first place.

Raw vs. Cooked: Nutrient Loss?

In various modern dieting communities — carnivore, primal, raw paleo, and more — there is a big debate about raw vs. cooked meat. There are decent arguments for both sides, and everyone has their own preference.

For you, cooked may seem like the only option at this point. Others may want to experiment with raw. Or you may get to a point where you want to vary it depending upon the specific food.

There is one important factor in all of this though. Our ancestors consumed food raw, cooked, and fermented. There was never a group of people who focused on one of these specifically and abandoned all the rest. And this was part of how they got nutrition, particularly in terms of using fermented food for Vitamin K2 (and just preservation before refrigeration).

On the raw side, some people do it just to feel more like a caveman. Others are worried about degrading the nutrient content by cooking. But when it comes to considering vitamins and minerals, as I have said a million times by now, the constant is the food quality. This is what's important.

Yes, braising a chunk of beef for one hour will cause it to lose some of its B vitamins. They may even be cut in half depending upon the method, time, and type of meat. You could even lose all of the Vitamin C with longer preparation times, and there is a possibility of reducing even some of the fat-soluble vitamins. (There are certainly enzymes and bacteria that are altered as well, but unfortunately there isn't much data on this.)

But this won't be much of a concern for anybody who — like most of us meat eaters — cooks their steak to rare or even medium. Rather than worrying about losing a few percentage points of your vitamin content, start by getting high-quality meat to begin with. The nutrient profile of feedlot beef is suspect to begin with. So you're better off eating a few ounces of a freshly slaughtered, fatty steak raised on summer pasture that was cooked all the way to well done than choking down four pounds of grain-fed poison raw.

One last thing to know is that freezing and storage time can affect the nutrient content. Vitamin C, especially, will be lost the longer you wait after the animal is killed. Some other nutrients, perhaps Vitamin B, can be affected. But as long as you aren't eating meat that is months upon months old, you will probably not be losing all that much.

Chapter Ten

Understanding Natural Hunger: The Three Types of Satiety

After becoming a full-time carnivore, I began to understand a few things about hunger. Some days, I am just not that hungry. Other times I can eat pounds and pounds of steak in a single sitting.

As an experiment, I once spent some time following the typical YouTuber carnivore diet of nothing but grain-fed ribeye steaks. I was insatiable. I could just keep eating and eating until my stomach was physically stuffed.

I have long attributed this hunger signaling to my body's needs. When Frankie Boy needs more Vitamin A, I crave liver. If I haven't had any sun all week, it might be salmon. If I need energy, it's fat. That's why I think I could eat so much conventionally raised ribeye at once. Well-seasoned steak — while delicious — doesn't provide all the nutrition you need.

People who eat this way can feel great in comparison to the Standard American Diet (SAD). Low inflammation levels alone can make a huge difference for people who are used to being bloated and struggling to digest antinutrient-full plant foods. But it isn't sufficient.

Understanding How Real Hunger Really Works

A few years ago, it all clicked. Interestingly enough, I was making natural, raw milk ice cream at the time. The heavy cream was delicious, but I couldn't eat much of it.

I otherwise had been eating very well and knew I was fully stocked up on all my vitamins and nutrients. And after eating sufficient fat and protein, my energy needs were all met. As good as that ice cream tasted, my body just didn't want it. And now that I've been eating this way, I listen to my body. It's usually right.

Because this was homemade, Frankie Boy-style ice cream, it didn't resemble anything you would buy in a store. There was a little bit of raw honey, but even that paled in comparison with the tons of corn syrup they add in a factory, not to mention all the other crap.

Processed food is all about trickery. Modern culinary techniques used in ice cream — and, really, almost everything you find packaged — include adding crazy amounts of sweetness, flavorings, and additives in carefully researched ratios to create an artificial palatability. This fools you into eating when you don't want to (more money for them) by masking natural hunger signals. And because most of society has been eating this stuff for decades now, people lack the ability to stop eating junk or crave what they actually need.

It was around the time of my ice cream experiment that I started thinking more about real hunger. I soon began to consciously eat foods in a certain order most of the time when I sat down at the table. This method helps to make sure that our natural appetites match up with our nutritional needs. It is also how some researchers believe our ancestors ate.

When an animal was killed, the prized organs, especially the liver, probably would have been eaten first. This was followed by the fat and then — though not always — muscle meat. Little went to waste but if a predator lurked or weather threatened the hunter and something had to be left behind, it would be the "steak," not the liver or bone marrow.

If you eat this way, you will notice that there are different types of satiety. The most nutrient-dense foods usually satiate you fast. A few bites of salmon roe are all most people will want. Some people really do love the taste of liver, but even they probably won't want more than a few ounces.

Taste is part of this phenomenon. But this isn't all about palatability. Even foods widely seen as delicious — like egg yolks and bone marrow — have a potency and richness that typically make people naturally unable to eat them in bulk.

Fat has a different level of satiety. Try eating raw butter. Especially if you eat a Keto Diet or a Carnivore Diet and run on a fat metabolism, it will taste great. Two tablespoons is probably plenty though. It may start to make you nauseous if you keep trying to gulp down any more. Few people will truly want to go back for five spoonfuls.

Eating grass-fed, slightly charred beef fat is more delicious. I can eat a lot more fat that a cow stored on its body than liver, butter, or even marrow, a food that I simply love. But fat will also start to become less palatable before long. You can even get nauseous from this too. And as long as you have been eating well in recent weeks and months, this will probably happen before your stomach is bulging.

The same even goes for cheese — a very highly palatable food. But you will notice that raw, grass-fed cheeses tend to be much richer and taste heavier than the store-bought "cheeses" that you have had in the past on deli sandwiches or nachos. Those products were designed by corporations to be extra palatable (by using "natural" flavoring) and entice people to eat more and more. Classic cheeses — think bleu Roquefort and Parmigiano-Reggiano — have enough of a funk and character that they taste great but satiate you much faster.

The Hunger for Fat vs. The Hunger for Protein

As delicious as cheese and certain fats can be, there is still usually some hunger signals that prompt you to stop eating. This is partly because digesting fat requires bile, a substance made in limited quantities in your gallbladder.

So while your appetite for carbs and protein is mostly just an issue of stomach size, fat simply cannot be handled by your system in massive volume. And your body will know this at some level even if your tongue does not.

Muscle meat, on the other hand, does not come with the same hunger type of signaling. Raw meat may lose its palatability quicker. But you can still eat a lot. And if it is well cooked on the grill with some salt — and then you add some black pepper or mustard sauce or balsamic vinegar — there may be no end to how much you can eat. Not consuming enough fat can also result in consuming excess protein.

For protein, satiation is also more dependent on lean body mass. A bodybuilder or an athlete with a high muscle mass will likely eat significantly more protein than the average person.

Eating for Your Natural Appetite

Knowing these three different types of satiety is key to understanding our natural appetite. On some level — and especially the further you are away from eating processed and sugar-loaded crap — our bodies know what they need. This is why I recommend regularly doing something of a "meal test" to calibrate your hunger and give your body exactly what it needs.

Start by eating the most nutrient-dense part of the meal. Liver, other organs, fish roe, marrow, eggs. Have a few bites of whatever food you are using as the primary means of getting in your daily nutrition. If you have any vitamin or other nutrient deficiencies, your appetite for these foods may change day to day.

Some people will simply never like liver. I am neutral on the taste but will admit that I don't love it. Even those who loathe it, though, should have more tolerance for it when Vitamin A levels are lower. Over time, your mind and gut learn to work together to make that connection. Your body will start to associate certain foods with certain nutrients. The Standard American Diet has destroyed this natural ability within most people, but it is something you can reestablish with patience and time. You might end up being amazed. In just a few weeks, you might find yourself craving a food that you hate.

After eating the most nutrient-dense food to satiety, move on to the main fatty part of the meal. For me, this is usually straight fat from a ruminant animal, usually beef or lamb. Other people may use grass-fed dairy or simply high-fat cuts of meat, but ideally the fat will be separate from the main protein portion. The fat will serve two main purposes: adding even more nutrients (animals store many vitamins and minerals in their fat) and supplying energy through calories.

Finally, move on to the protein. This should have the lowest satiety level, so it is best to eat last after you have already fulfilled your bigger needs from other sources. You will then reach your protein demand and likely continue eating beyond that for more calories. If you weren't that hungry to begin with, you may stop before long.

Other times, you might eat until your stomach starts to physically feel full. With meat, you still likely won't get that massive bloated and distended feeling that comes from eating a whole pizza or bag of Doritos. But your stomach has a certain capacity and the meat could start to approach it. Still, you probably won't completely stuff yourself on steak if you're not drowning it in salt, pepper, or sauces that make it unnaturally palatable.

You do not have to eat this way every single time you sit down at the table. And you don't have to eat organ meats every day. Generally, on a daily basis, I personally enjoy eating fat first then alternating between protein and fat until I've reached full satiety. But it can certainly help to do this meal test several times.

The more you do these meal tests, the more you will reset your natural appetite and learn about the different levels of hunger and different types of satiety. In time, this will retrain your mind, stomach, and body to understand when, what, and how much you should be eating.

Our evolution created the hormones in our gut and mind. Learning how they work — and how they signal appetite — will make it much easier to eat for nutrient density and optimal health.

Chapter Eleven

FAQ: Addressing Common Ancestral Indigenous Diet Concerns

With any diet, new adopters are going to have some questions. The same applies with the Indigenous Ancestral Diet. It's only natural to have some confusion about a nutrition-based philosophy that is so different from everything you have always been taught.

Really, it isn't that complicated. There are some staple foods — specifically, high-quality animal foods — that you will start eating a lot. And there will be many other things you once thought were healthy that will no longer enter your mouth.

This knowledge is enough to get you started. Within a few weeks, you will begin to better understand the "why" of everything. As you feel better, you will start to realize that Frankie Boy might just be onto something here. This should motivate you to commit harder.

That's one great part about these philosophies. Even incorporating a few tips will help a lot. Then, the sky's the limit. You will get as much out of it as you put in.

That said, it won't be a seamless transition. I have covered most of the fundamentals already. But I wanted to take this extra time here to try to answer some of the most frequently asked questions (FAQs) about the Ancestral Indigenous Diet.

How will I feel at the beginning? Is there an adaptation period, and how difficult is the transition?

I won't lie. I actually had a hard time adjusting to this diet. It took me months to get it right. But that was because I realized that I simply wasn't eating enough fat. I spent my whole life in a fat-phobia world and I guess it must have even rubbed off on me.

After incorporating some bison fat into my diet, and eating according to my natural appetite, I started feeling great literally within a matter of days. It was that easy. Don't make the same mistake. Eat plenty of fat.

Otherwise, the transition to feeling much better can happen quite quickly. And you now have the benefit of all the experience and knowledge that Frankie the Guinea Pig learned through trial and error. If everything is done properly, there shouldn't be more than a period of a few days of feeling anything negative. (This will last two weeks at the very most.)

The main problems people have are related to not eating enough fat (throwing off your fat-to-protein ratio) or not getting enough nutrients. (The most common things I see are people not getting enough Vitamin A, usually because they are not eating liver, or Vitamin D3, due to lack of sunlight or proper supplementation.) Secondary issues can come up due to allergies to certain foods or a histamine intolerance, which can generally be recognized fairly easily.

The adaptation period could also be more difficult for anyone suffering from more severe damage to their gut and overall health due to years of eating a terrible diet or other individual factors. In general, this diet will make you healthier and is not just safe but overwhelmingly beneficial for almost everyone.

But the stress of change — especially psychologically — on top of an already over-stressed body can be hard for some people. As always, monitor your own health, watch for potential warning signs, and consult your doctor if you are concerned that you are responding especially poorly.

What about cholesterol and saturated fat? Won't I have a heart attack if all I eat is meat?

The war over cholesterol has been waging for years and shows no signs of ending anytime soon. The same goes for different types of fats. Detailing it all would take an entire book, so it is not something I can cover in depth here. But the principles of this diet are rooted in the notion that ancient humans ate high-fat, animal-based diets for tens of thousands of years and lived largely free from degenerative diseases, including heart disease.

To the degree that health industry bogeymen like saturated fat and cholesterol can be linked to heart problems, it is my belief that this is largely all wrapped up in the larger problem of inflammation. This is the true culprit in most aspects of our negative health. More and more evidence is showing that sugar and modern processed food are what is poisoning us from within. Specific to heart disease, the combination of high carbohydrate diets and vegetable seed oils are the driving causes. Each disease we suffer from as humans has a specific cause, which is camouflaged by the illusion of what we've been told our whole lives. By understanding the functions in the body associated with any issues you are having, you can address the root cause.

While some people who follow a carnivore diet long-term do have cholesterol panels that may seem alarming by conventional standards, the fact that this way of eating greatly reduces inflammation means that there is little to worry about. This is what I believe based upon combing through endless studies and research on the topic over the years.

Consultations with doctors are always advisable if you don't feel well. But eating high-quality animal foods will make you and your heart healthier — not worse. More up-to-date medical doctors will look at much more than just cholesterol, examining inflammatory markers, blood sugar, and triglycerides, for instance.

How many cheat days do I get? How strict do I have to be?

Most diets you read about in a book advocate moderation and give you the flexibility to go crazy once in awhile. But this diet really is a way of achieving excellent health. There is no built-in room for cheating.

Clearly, you will not go the rest of your entire life without having a few bad foods that you once enjoyed. Most people will have some alcohol here and there as well. But the goal here is health — not simply weight loss or some short-term benefit — and every time you stray from the path, it is a step in the wrong direction.

That said, there is a big difference between putting some sauce on your steak vs. eating a slice of pizza. It's also important to know that certain preparation methods — as with sour dough bread or homemade ice cream from high-quality dairy — will allow you to enjoy some foods that should never be consumed in their store-bought form. Granted, sourcing these ingredients can get expensive, and the preparation required is far more laborious than stopping by an ice cream parlor for 10 minutes.

That said, few people are monks and there will be slip ups. So any time you are going to consume something that you know is negative for your health, the first consideration should be tolerance. If you are allergic or have low-level inflammatory reactions to the food, then the damage to your gut may be too great to risk your health goals. Think about it like this: Eating excess calories — and thus impairing weight loss — is not as big of an issue as eating something that will cause gut microbiome imbalances.

If you are cheating, try to stick to minimally inflammatory alternatives you are not allergic to. Do you really need that slice of pie or can you just over-eat steak or macadamia nuts and get through this bad day? Would some harmful, but not disastrous, chicken wings get you through this urge? Consider actual bad foods a last resort if emotional stress or lack of sleep leaves you feeling like you have to stuff yourself.

It's important to realize if a craving is psychological or an actual craving. In most cases, this is also a temporary issue at the start of the adaptation period that will pass in time. Beyond two to three weeks of strict dieting, cravings that were once rooted in a carb withdrawal will start to go away. Any remaining cravings will likely be related to micronutrient deficiency (eat some liver or cheese and get some sun) or macronutrient deficiency, a lack of protein or energy calories in the diet (fat or carbohydrate).

Ultimately, consistently consuming high-nutrient foods — like organ meats, wild-caught fish, and salmon roe — along with enough high-quality fat will ensure you are satiated. You will operate on a fat-based metabolism and not find yourself panicking for the comfort foods of your past in between your large, satiating meals. You will stop being hungry for "cheat meals."

The biggest temptations will then come from social situations. With enough self confidence and belief in the principles of this way of eating, you will be able to control yourself and not end up snacking on potato chips just to fit in with the crowd. For extra motivation, just glance around to remind yourself how sickly most people look. You can live and feel better than that. If you want to.

What about mercury and ocean pollution? Should I really be eating seafood?

It's pretty rich to hear people who regularly eat Taco Bell, microwave lasagna, and "tofurkey" laboratory concoctions stay away from Alaskan salmon and oysters because they are worried about their health.

Yeah, the ocean is definitely dirty. And these fish are likely quite a bit worse in quality than they were even just a century ago. But they are still real food with real nutrition — not inflammatory calorie bombs that offer up no legitimate benefits like most of the stuff people eat every day.

Heavy metal toxicity really isn't a concern with the fatty fish and shellfish I am recommending. Species very high on the food chain, like shark and swordfish, can potentially present more problems. And eating wild-caught salmon at every single meal may be pushing it.

But having enough seafood each week to help meet your DHA needs, in lieu of brains and dozens upon dozens of eggs, is probably not going to fill your blood with mercury or otherwise cause any real problem.

If you are truly scared, what can I say? The important part really is just to get your Omega 3s in. If you want to only dine on sardines and lamb brains instead, be my guest. But we need this stuff to live — and algae and flaxseed oil will not get the job done.

What the crap? Won't I be constipated constantly without any fiber?

Not quite. All of our indigenous ancestors consumed fiber in some form. Some consumed a lot, some maybe once per year. But it has no necessary function in our diets, and believe it or not, you will not have any bowel or constipation issues due to a lack of fiber.

Different foods digest at different rates. When we consume only meat our digestion rate slows, as meat and fat (animal foods) digest very slowly compared to plant foods. This is because the body absorbs far more nutrition and it takes time to extract it.

So before you get worried, ask yourself this: Are you actually constipated, meaning stuff down there is uncomfortable? Or are you just going to the bathroom less? You will likely continue not going to the toilet as often as you used to — and that is not a problem. If there isn't any discomfort involved, it probably isn't actually constipation. (And consider troubleshooting your water and hydration levels as well. Meat probably won't be the problem when it comes to digestion.)

Actual digestive problems that arise on this diet usually can be traced to three possibilities: food quality, cooking temperature, and cross contamination.

If you're consuming high-Omega-6 food (like poor-quality pork), it might not digest well at all. If the fat you consume is overcooked (heavily rendered), the body may not be able to produce enough enzymes and bile to properly break it all down and this often results in diarrhea. If the meat has harmful bacteria from cross contamination introduced during processing, that can obviously create significant issues in the gut.

Again, the ratio of fat to protein should not be ignored, as too much of either will put stress on digestion. You may experience some issues at the beginning as you transition. But most people, within a few weeks, report feeling better in their gut than they ever have. Inflammation is largely removed and you will finally be digesting — and crapping — as nature intended.

What about coffee? Yeah, it comes from a plant, but I can still drink it, right?

No. I have never drank coffee — nor have I ever needed coffee. For me Vitamin D3 has always been my energy booster. You should avoid it too. The reason we want to eliminate it is because of the anti-nutrient content, in the form of phytic acid, that can potentially harm our absorption of minerals. Coffee is also just inflammatory in general, and caffeine stresses the adrenals, something that can be more of a problem for women.

Of course, I know many people won't give this up. You should at least try to limit consumption though, and one alternative is espresso (or an "Americano," which is an espresso with extra hot water added). Because the brew time is quicker, the water has less exposure to the beans and this means it has fewer anti-nutrients. It also has less caffeine despite its reputation as a pick-me-up. Tea is also another option that is probably better in most cases.

Will I develop allergies? What are the signs? And what are histamines?

One of the best parts about this the Ancestral Indigenous Diet is that it serves as an "elimination diet." You mainly will be eating a limited menu of items that will expand in time as you improve your food sourcing ability. And this will make it relatively easy to identify any foods that are introduced and cause poor reactions.

What is a poor reaction? What are you looking for? If you've been living with high levels of inflammation for years — or decades — it may be tougher to identify at first. Acute allergies should be relatively easy to spot. Whether it's digestive problems, gas, skin breakouts, or more severe issues like nausea or vomiting, you will know it when it happens.

Another issue may be a histamine response from high-histamine foods. We see this most often with aged and fermented foods such as cheese, yogurt, sauerkraut, kimchi, pickles, kombucha, or cured meats. Alcohol and vinegar are common culprits. So are seemingly safe items like frozen/salted/canned fish, citrus, or even egg whites. Common histamine side effects are headaches, congestion, fatigue, hives, digestive issues, nausea, vomiting, and heart palpitations.

Histamine is an organic nitrogen compound that may trigger an allergic response in human and mammalian systems. Other biogenic amines such as cadaverine are contained in certain foods as well. When a food ages, as most meats we eat has for many weeks, the histamine content increases. When you are consuming mostly animal foods, this increased histamine load causes issues in a certain percentage of people.

One cause of histamine intolerance lies within the body's ability, or lack thereof, to produce histamine-removing enzymes, hypothetically from a lack of certain nutrients. The more common cause is dysbiosis (a gut bacterial imbalance), resulting in more histamine-producing bacteria in your stomach, as opposed to histamine-degrading bacteria.

It seems like a simple problem to fix. Restore nutrients and fix the microbiome. And that does work for many. But to fix the microbiome you generally have to consume high-histamine probiotic foods, so it needs to be addressed carefully on an individual basis.

Can I follow the Ancestral Indigenous Diet without a gallbladder?

Yes, you can make this work without a gallbladder. Initially, your body will have to adapt to a higher fat intake and you should be careful to not go overboard. In general, adjusting away from carbs might require more frequent meals of lower volumes of fat compared to higher-protein intake.

But, yes, you can still live — and thrive — on a nutrient-dense, animal-food diet. Be careful and look for warning signs of problems if you think your digestion is not working properly. Just know that there are many people following a high-fat diet, both ketogenic and carnivore, without a gallbladder and they do just fine.

Chapter Twelve

Beyond Nutrition: Water, Sleep, Sun, Exercise, and Modern Problems

Clever readers may remember that this book is called the Ancestral Indigenous Diet. So it should go without saying that the primary goal is to help you eat in a natural way. This is the biggest factor in getting as close as possible to your optimal health.

But it would be incomplete to focus solely on food. Frankie Boy has much more wisdom about health to share, and there are several other factors that you must consider in your daily life if you want to hit that goal.

Paying close attention to these areas can be particularly helpful when it comes to troubleshooting. If you think you are already eating perfectly but continue to have health issues, your problem might be solved by fixing stuff outside the kitchen.

The four other areas you need to understand are: water, exercise, sun exposure, and sleep. Our ancestors living long ago didn't really have to worry about any of these.

Well, water was likely always an issue — but only in terms of finding it and boiling it. Beyond some naturally occurring bugs and parasites, their water would have been clean and unaffected by the modern contaminants that are almost unavoidable today.

As in the rest of the book, that is the general theme here: We may have it easy living in modern society in many ways, but our new problems are subtly destroying our health. Unfortunately, in today's modern world, these once-customary elements of life have become a lot more complicated. From artificial pollutants and sedentary desk work to sunburns and insomnia, we are dealing with a lot of issues that are relatively new in human history.

I won't go in depth on any of these factors for simplicity's sake. You do need to pay close attention to each of them though. Because they intersect with your diet in very important ways, and it is impossible to truly feel your best without getting them all right. Even after getting your diet on point, you will have to overcome modern pitfalls in a few other key areas if you want to achieve natural, ancestral health.

Water

Just about everyone would agree that staying hydrated is important. It is one of the three essential components of life. One old adage says that a person can survive three weeks without food, three days without water, and three minutes without air.

Even though everyone understands this, most people still give little thought to what water they are drinking. We are taught to hydrate — eight glasses a day — and replenish electrolytes after exercise. But consuming chemical contaminants like fluoride (which they say is good for your teeth) or chlorine (which they use to remove bacteria) is far from what nature intended.

This is made even worse by the other substances found in modern water. Aging plumbing, pollution, and other factors means that are taps water may have both physical problems (measured in parts per million, or PPM, as total dissolved solids like lead, other heavy metals, and various toxins) and chemical problems (including those mentioned above as well as antibiotics, pesticides, and herbicides).

Fluoride may be associated with brain damage, reduced IQ, impaired ability to learn and remember, and impaired fetal brain development. Chlorine, like flouride, can block iodine receptors and in high doses may be a toxic chemical with links to heart attacks, asthma, and organ damage. Pharmaceuticals like birth control can disrupt hormones. Other toxins and chemicals cause oxidative stress. And, across the board, we need to worry about various herbicides, pesticides, and antibiotics.

Many people are well aware of how dirty municipal water supplies have become. But turning to bottled water often isn't a great solution. Often, there are other problems introduced from plastic leaching from bottles that sit in the sun and heat for hours on a pallet.

Mineral water in glass bottles from good (often European) sources can be a good option. But this becomes expensive and unrealistic for most people on an everyday basis. That said, transitioning to glass bottles for a few weeks can be a good experiment. If you try this and notice an improvement in your energy levels and how you feel overall, it may mean that your previous water sources may be inadequate and you need to take more extreme actions.

The sad reality in modern society is that we can only go so far in some cases when it comes to optimizing our water source. The best advice is to start by doing an in-home test (kits are available on Amazon) and, if necessary, install an in-home filtration system. The time and money you invest is almost always worth it.

A more in-depth look at all this can be found on my YouTube channel, and it is definitely easier to follow a video "How To" explanation about filtration. But most people will do very well by installing a reverse-osmosis filter. It is relatively easy to set up and very affordable — especially when you consider how much it will help your health. Reverse osmosis and distillation still may not remove all the chemical and antibiotic concerns, but the water will still be infinitely better than anything straight out of the tap.

By removing a large amount of the physical and chemical impurities, you will be greatly reducing potential inflammation (including the destruction of gut bacteria), any electrolyte imbalance (due to an incorrect mineral profile of water), and generally optimizing your hydration. This way, you can be confident that you are consuming something that has a net positive impact.

After quality comes the question of quantity. Do we really need eight glasses per day? Should we follow the gymrats who pound water by the gallon? Are we OK being like our ancestors who may have consumed less in times of scarcity?

If we look to the past, there was wide variation in how much water people consumed. This was largely dependent upon geographical and environmental factors. People in deserts may have often consumed very little water, and we know that groups like the Maasai in Kenya have a tradition of drinking blood from livestock. This is now mainly a ceremonial ritual, but anthropologists have long seen evidence of this practice in many cultures, often in dry climates.

Other indigenous groups in areas of abundance have consumed large volumes of water. This is true both among some that have lived near large aquifers or cold locations with lots of snowfall.

In a natural human sense, there may be no exact set amount to consume for optimal health. Even today, many people consider hydration to be fairly personal. This is likely just something you will want to experiment with. If you feel better with high volumes, that could be perfect for you. If you start to feel lethargic, you might be drinking too much water and peeing out more electrolytes than you are consuming. And all this can be affected by how much salt and other electrolytes you consume with your food.

My advice is to figure out what works for you and stick with it. Consistency and individual requirements will be something you can dial in over time. It may seem a little complicated at first. But as the rest of your nutrition becomes better, your body will start to give you better signals about how much it needs.

Exercise

We know that our ancient ancestors got a lot more physical activity than we do today. Even just at the start of the 1900s, the majority of people were still working the fields, physically doing construction, or otherwise spending most of the day on their feet. And this of course likely pales in comparison to the near-constant activity early humans performed when it came to hunting, looking for water, or living a nomadic lifestyle.

Today, most people spend all day sitting at a desk or in a car, struggling to find even an hour to go get some exercise. While this is unfortunate and our modern sedentary existence is certainly contributing to some of our health problems, too many people look at working out as a means to lose weight and make up for a bad diet.

People run on a treadmill because our society's ingrained preconceived notions tell us that cardio is the path to weight loss. New fads push 5x5 powerlifting routines to gain muscle mass. In general, exercise and resistance training is a heavily goal-dependent activity. But most people just follow the masses and fail to achieve anything, let alone ever cut the belly fat or unleash the hypertrophy they need to add lean muscle.

As a teenager and young adult, II was in the gym lifting for two hours a day, almost every day, for nearly 10 years. I gave that up when I realized I didn't even want to be a high-level bodybuilder. More importantly, I came to understand that the lifestyle wasn't making me happy — or helping my health at all.

But I am glad that the experience taught me about the importance of building up muscle mass. Even though following this diet will promote an increase in muscle mass even without working out — simply by consuming so much high-quality animal food — it will help to incorporate some resistance training.

With a proper, high-volume routine, you can add muscle even without lifting super heavy weights. You will also fix postural and musculoskeletal imbalances created by our sedentary lives without putting massive strain on your ligaments, tendons, and central nervous system, all of which can become overstressed by extended cardio work or powerlifting programs.

You can also just make an effort to walk more often. Skip lunch and take a long, hour-long walk three times a week on your break from work. It may do more good than hiring a personal trainer. Better yet, start hiking. The fresh air and uphill walks on the weekend closely resemble how most ancient humans likely spent much of their day.

At the end of the day, we are physical beings. While living a modern life, most of us will never be as active as our ancestral indigenous forefathers. And we will never have access to the same pristine streams for our water or truly wild game living on unpolluted, naturally pure pasture.

You still need to do all you can though. And while ancient peoples built their lean muscle mass by building shelters, tracking game, and carrying their kill back home, we need to put things up and put them down in a Planet Fitness. It isn't an evolutionarily ideal situation. But just a little bit of effort in the gym or hiking on a trail will help you get closer to your ideal health. Most people see their body composition improve after a few months on the carnivore diet, putting on significant muscle while losing excess body fat.

Sun

By now, after reading about the fundamentals of the Ancestral Indigenous Diet, you should already know how important Vitamin D3 is for your health. And you know that getting some sun is the best way to hit your optimal levels. So let me start off here by offering another personal anecdote about my attempts to get enough sunshine.

Years ago, during a time when I was waiting tables at Del Frisco's steakhouse in New York, I had developed a slight sunburn after laying out for about 15 hours in two days. To help heal, I decided to rub cod liver oil on my skin. But I was entirely unaware of just how *awful* it smelled. All of the other waiters started asking people if they could smell some foul fish. Where was this coming from?

I was exhausted from working too many hours at the time, so I didn't really care. But in hindsight, it must have been *terrible*. So just a quick piece of advice: Whatever you do, don't use cod liver oil as a balm if you overdo your time outside.

That may just be a Frankie problem though. Most other people are much more concerned about skin cancer or thinking that they will always burn if they get too much UV exposure.

But you need to consider several things. One is that humans have historically adjusted to increased sunlight over the course of the year. We wouldn't have run out directly to the beach after spending six straight months in a cave. In more northern and far southern latitudes, we would have been outside often throughout the year, so the sporadic April and May rays would start to get us prepared — as our skin darkens with more melatonin — for the long, direct summer UV levels.

Second is that our modern diets make sunburns more of a problem. Specifically, the unnaturally high Omega-6 to Omega-3 ratios cause inflammation, which doesn't allow our bodies to properly heal our skin after extended exposure and prevent it from being damaged.

Because I prioritize tanning in the summer months, I do occasionally overdo it. There may be an amazing day in late May when I haven't yet built up any base and I spend an extra hour laying out. But any initial bit of pinkness I see will disappear entirely by morning and turn to brown. This is because my system is always full of adequate nutrition and is never subject to the chronic inflammation that prevents most people today from allowing their immune system to quickly take care of a minor issue like a small sunburn.

Understanding this really shouldn't take much of a leap in logic. Is it really possible that our ancient ancestors were unable to spend even two or three hours a day out in the sun? Because nowadays, there are many people who won't even consider leaving their house in July without long sleeves, a big hat, and cream all over their face. If humans were this delicate throughout our history, we never would have made it.

They probably weren't damaged by even long sun exposure because they maintained a great Omega ratio and stores of fat-soluble vitamins, particularly Vitamin A, which is the most important vitamin for healing tissue (and the one so many people lack today).

You should of course be smart about sun exposure. There is no need to overdo it. Moderate exposure everyday is better than one 10-hour session that fries you once per week.

In general, the required dosage of Vitamin D3 is dependent on the immediate need. Have you been deficient your whole life? Do you live somewhere that allows you to get Vitamin D3 all year long? Are you a pregnant or nursing woman? Do you have skin conditions that might be caused by a Vitamin D3 deficiency?

Depending upon the answers to these and other questions, you should adjust how much sun you get. The best idea is to just get sun when you can. And you can start with a blood-level test to see where you are starting from.

If it's been raining for a week straight and Sunday turns out to be a sunny day, skip going to the movies and hit the park. Same goes for lunchtime at work if the sun starts shining. Get out there and soak in some UVB for an hour while you can.

And anyone who, like me, lives in a place like New York where significant exposure is almost impossible for half the year, do your best to stock up stores during the summer. Then, you will be in better shape by the time Halloween rolls around and can get by with some supplementation or tanning beds until it's spring again.

Sleep

You don't need me to tell you about the importance of sleep. You've been hearing it your whole life. Chances are, you still aren't getting enough, and I won't be able to convince you to start changing things now.

You're already supposed to eat a bunch of strange foods and cut out many of your favorites. Now I'm expecting you to go from six hours a night to the recommended amount? Good luck with that, buddy.

Well, you know what? I'm going to say it anyway: You should get more sleep. But there are a few other aspects beyond the duration that matter as well, and maybe you'll listen about these.

For starters, you get your 8 hours of sleep per night and you're good-to-go, right? Maybe not. Why do most people — even those lucky few who are getting enough sleep — feel awful? It might be about the quality of the sleep itself.

To be completely honest, as a long-time bartender I should probably be the last person giving sleeping advice. But as someone who has struggled most of their life to get enough rest, there are definitely things that work, and a lot of them tie into natural sleeping patterns.

There is a lot of research into circadian rhythms and how light patterns affect our ability to get good, quality, restorative sleep no matter how many hours it lasts. But one interesting piece of information came a few years ago from *National Geographic*.

They visited several modern indigenous tribes — the Tsimane of the Bolivian Amazon, the Hadza society of Tanzania, and the San people in Namibia — who still live without electricity and artificial light to see how they slept.

Unlike a popular hypothesis, they didn't necessarily get more sleep than us city and suburbia dwellers. But their sleeping habits did tend to match their local environment.

"Though the San, Tsimane, and Hadza often average less than seven hours of sleep, they seem to be getting enough sleep," wrote journalist Traci Watson. "They seldom nap, and they don't have trouble dozing off. The San and Tsimane languages have no word for insomnia, and when researchers tried to explain it to them, 'they still don't seem to quite understand.'"

While the scientific data and anecdotal evidence like this is often conflicting and confusing when it comes to sleep duration, everyone seems to agree that getting quality sleep is the most important.

One way to improve this is by blacking out your room. Especially if you have been chronically exhausted, sleeping in a pitch black room and letting your body wake up naturally — as opposed to being disturbed by the brightness of the sun — may help you reset your natural sleep needs.

Everyone, and especially people who have trouble falling asleep, should also seek to reduce blue light at night. This light, which is emitted from modern screens, including phones, can inhibit the production of melatonin (our sleep hormone) and generally confuse the body about the natural light patterns that should trigger tiredness.

Beyond everything else, you should hopefully see improvement just due to a better diet. Your hormones and energy levels will be more stable and better regulated once you get your vitamins and nutrients in check. This alone, plus a little bit more physical activity during the day, should have you sleeping deeper and in a more natural way even within a few weeks.

Chapter Thirteen

Eating as Nature Intended: Your Journey to Optimal Health

There are hundreds of other aspects of diet that I have either not mentioned or only briefly touched on in this book. The bogeyman of cholesterol is one prime example. This is because, honestly, that could be an entire book in and of itself, and the science and studies needed to get into everything are vast.

In short, you can generally just walk away knowing that high-quality plant foods do have more cholesterol than the standard American diet but that is not a problem you need to worry about because inflammation — as we discussed in an entire chapter — is the real killer when it comes to heart disease.

Then there is protein. You may be shocked by how little that was even mentioned here. Coming from a bodybuilding background, a world where protein intake is the only thing anyone cares about, I am all too aware of how much this is discussed in most nutritional conversations. Really, most of the popular diet recommendations over the past few decades have always focused heavily on one of the three macronutrients. One is always a big problem area while the others are the best thing since sliced bread.

While I didn't speak about it that much, yes, carbs are the odd man out here in the Ancestral Indigenous Diet. But it is not in the same sense as, say, the Keto Diet or the Atkins Diet. Instead, the lack of carbs in the Ancestral Indigenous Diet is more the natural result of focusing on high-quality foods (which come from animals) and staying away from all inflammation and anti-nutrients (which is mostly coming from carb-heavy modern plant foods and processed junk).

Protein, on the other hand, is absolutely essential. But if you eat along with the principles I explained in this book, focusing on protein intake is not actually important. Because if you're aiming for nutrient density and now understand where that comes from, your protein intake will inherently be met. Make sure you follow me: Protein is very important, but focusing on consuming it is not — when following this diet — because you will get enough naturally. In fact, my main mistake early on when I started eating this way was consuming too much protein. Or, more accurately, I was not consuming enough fat, and I was lacking energy because of that.

Another area you might be wondering about is electrolytes, especially if you've been spending time on keto forums where they talk about Lite Salt and Snake Juice all day long. Or what about calories in, calories out and visceral vs. subcutaneous fat? Why didn't Frankie talk about insulin spikes, the glycemic index, and ketones? Where do I get my antioxidants, polyphenols, and flavanols? Shouldn't I be consuming apple cider vinegar, green tea, and dark chocolate? Don't I need prebiotics, probiotics, and resistant starch to keep my gut healthy?

Humans tend to overcomplicate things. They isolate specifics and analyze them to death. But in most cases, nature has a more reasonable answer.

Some more granular questions are indeed intriguing and new science continues to show us some interesting things (although less than most magazines would have you believe). I myself have spent hours researching findings about mechanisms like the Krebs cycle, mineral chelation, stomach acid concentrations, sodium-potassium exchange, and the hormetic effects of various things we consume.

A lot of these details, however, are really just distractions for the average person. If you are LeBron James and eating a perfect diet and you need to get that one extra 0.001% of performance, some of these things on the margins might be worth pursuing. Any possible means of improving ATP and mitochondrial function would be worth exploring.
Even the average person can experiment here and there by seeing how their gut responds to A1 vs A2 milk. I have often tried different things, from eating seaweed to putting clay in my water, to find an ideal balance of electrolytes. And I have played around with raw honey, consuming small servings before exercise to see if it has any effect on performance.

You need to be realistic though. Most people eat like shit. And they've been eating like shit for decades. Even those of use who think we're doing everything right — like Frankie Boy back when he was a sculpted bodybuilder hitting the gym everyday like a good boy — are still mostly ingesting poison and inflammatory garbage that provides very few nutrients.

So that's what you need to focus on. Get the nutrition that you now understand is essential. Cut out the crap that is leaving you inflamed and destroying your digestive system. Keep finding better and better sources of high-quality food now that you actually know what that means. And work to improve all of the other stuff — water, exercise, sun, and sleep — that we all have always known is important to health.

Then, once you do all that, *maybe* — and I do mean *maybe* — you could start researching some studies and wondering if green tea really is beneficial. (It probably isn't.) You could try seeing if wild blueberry antioxidants do anything for you. (They definitely aren't necessary.) Or, screw it, even try out some fancy hipster mushrooms for whatever purported benefits people think they might have. (Who even knows?)

As I stated at the beginning of this book, I try to always remain open minded. I have said time and time again here in this book (and almost daily on my YouTube channel) that every indigenous group has consumed some plant foods, often as one-third of their diet (by caloric intake). So while I am a carnivore and see little value in eating most modern plant foods when calories are no longer scarce, there very well may be some case to be made for certain plant foods when it comes to areas like feeding the gut microbiome.

We are only now starting to really understand how the digestive system works. Who knows? We may even still find out that polyphenols or other micronutrients really do have some benefits that make them worth consuming. But the evidence is still spurious at best.

And some things are certain. I do know, for example, that the vast — vast — majority of Americans are not getting enough Vitamin A, Vitamin D3, or Vitamin K2. I am positive that all the seed oils, soy-fed chicken breast, and deli ham slices are ruining their Omega fatty acid ratios. And I know that inflammation is killing people, destroying families, and keeping millions of people hooked on pharmaceuticals that they would never have needed if they just ate like their great grandparents once did.

What I would love to see is even more science on these aspects of our diet. These big-ticket items still never get talked about while Healthline.com and Time magazine pump out 50 articles a year about how much red wine is ideal for your health. (It's probably zero cups per year.)

In trying to get more data about exact nutrient content of various foods, I have looked long and hard. There is a German nutritional database that seems far superior to the USDA standard breakdowns for many foods, particularly when it comes to things like liver and offcuts that the Washington regulator knows nobody in the United States under 70 actually eats anymore.

But it is still very hard to find the precise measurements on the difference between the vitamins in grass-fed beef fat vs. feedlot beef fat. In blanket-statement terms in the United States, this wouldn't even do much good. Because the legal definition of marketing terms like "grass-fed," "free-range," and "pastured" doesn't actually tell you much about how the animal was raised.

What I want to know is how much Vitamin K2 is actually in different artisanal raw cheeses and how much Vitamin C is lost by freezing the meat from a freshly killed lamb for two months. How much DHA is actually in a chicken that lives outdoors and eats bugs all day compared to one raised in a poultry concentration camp never seeing the sun?

One of my goals is to start doing this myself if nobody else ever will. But it's expensive and takes a lot of effort. Plus, as mentioned, even with the best (real) grass-fed, humanely raised cows, there will be some variance in nutrients due to the pasture it was on and what time of year it was killed (because summer grass has that much more chlorophyll and cows, like us, produce more Vitamin D3 during times of peak UV).

These are the questions I'm curious about. And if people in positions of power actually cared about helping people be healthier, these are the types of questions we would maybe get answers to. Instead, this stuff is hardly studied. Because there is no money in it.

Meanwhile, we get new research about goji berries every few months. Twenty years ago, it was pomegranates — just when they were becoming a hot product on the market. Funny how that works. Now, we hear more and more about gluten all the time — not because celiac disease is a serious problem for a small percentage of people but because "gluten-free" is a new marketing term that global food manufacturers know sells more product. And just watch: There will be dozens of new studies released in the next two years about fake meat when anybody who has any understanding of how it's made can tell you right now that it's just soy-based slop.

Without putting on too much of a tinfoil hat, this is because industry is the biggest funder of nutritional studies. They are also conducted in ways that make things very difficult to isolate, with factors like healthy bias and self-reporting. How do you find out what effect eggs have on the heart when the subjects in the study are downing seed oils on the side and this is supposedly just part of the control group? The epidemiological approaches yield results, sure, but they are so clouded by lifestyle factors and poorly understood relative risk conclusions.

Even well-meaning academics who are unaffiliated with interests like Monsanto and Cargill have little interest in exploring the topics that I think can most help us perfect our diets. This isn't even necessarily because they are evil or paid shills. It's that they gravitate to areas where they think societal "impact" can be made. If they are actually trying to do good, they probably know that true pasture-raised pork is so uncommon that studying it is unlikely to actually help many people. Investing their small $20,000 grant on this won't make much difference in their eyes. By comparison, doing a study that helps confirm that the Impossible Burger is just repackaged and reprocessed junk food may actually steer millions of people away from it.

The sad part is that they are probably right. With all the abundance and wealth we have in this country, we could be moving toward a diet utopia where everyone can eat the best eggs and cheese humanity is capable of producing. But nobody is actually pushing for this. They are lining up for the new Popeye's chicken sandwich in record numbers and then telling themselves they'll go vegan for a week to make up for their "cheat meal."

It's depressing. Everyone wants to talk about diet and nutrition all day long. But none of the conversations they are having are the right conversations. In a world like this, it's hard not to feel like I am just yelling in a room full of empty chairs.

But I know that the principles of health I am promoting here are real. And I know that people who adopt this way of eating — and, maybe more importantly, this way of thinking about food in general — will become healthier. I have seen it in my sister and many clients who have asked for my help in turning their lives around.

So even if the best I can hope for is getting one percent of Americans to truly consider and understand food quality, that's still 3.3 million people! Hopefully just a few of you will take this all to heart and be able to get over your obesity issues, get off those prescription drugs, and get back in control of your health. In a few years — and hopefully a few months — maybe you will be able to do things that today are simply out of reach now because you are tired and feel like crap all the time.

That's my goal. There may be no way to turn back the clock and convince people that feedlot beef, soy, and chronic inflammation are a three-pronged fork being rammed into our society's chest. And it may be decades before we learn to overcome the conventional wisdom fallacies that have the whole world following nutrient-deficient vegans into the grave. Quality animal foods, especially in the United States, may just continue to get harder and harder to find.

But there are some encouraging signs. Everyone now knows that Omega 3s are important. Eat local and small farm meat share co-ops are gaining popularity. Raw and artisanal cheeses are now widely available at mainstream places like Whole Foods. Even the momentum we are seeing for carnivore and keto diets — albeit with sellout influencers in these areas pushing feedlot beef and processed garbage — is a good sign that things may be changing.

So I will continue to have some hope — even in a seemingly hopeless world.

More than anything, though, I know that any single individual can change their life for the better. It will require rethinking some things and having awkward conversations in social situations. But it is definitely very achievable and, I hope, I have given you a good blueprint to follow.

From my YouTube channel to this book to my meat company to dreams of owning a farm and venturing out into various other areas of health, I know I am just getting started.

Hopefully, you can too. That's all it takes. Just get started on this journey to better health through a nutrient-dense, Ancestral Indigenous Diet, and you will be very happy you did.

So I will leave you with that.

Above all, I want you to be healthy and avoid so many of the problems that too many people now face. So many of these issues really are avoidable. All you have to do is eat like humans should.

More than anything else, if you want to start improving your future and feeling better in the present, you need to look to our past. The ancestral indigenous way of living may have had plenty of drawbacks. But when it comes to diet and health, they knew a lot of things that we have somehow forgotten as a society.

If you learn to rediscover your past, you will start to discover your health.

Printed in Great Britain
by Amazon